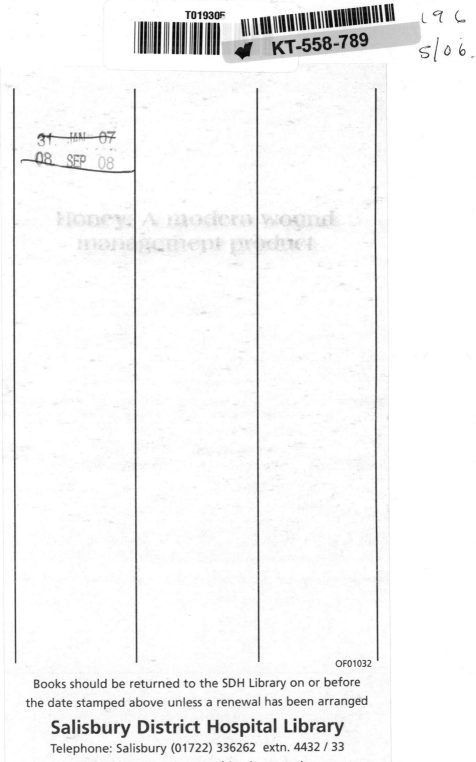

Other titles available from Wounds UK include:

A Pocket Guide to Clinical Decision Making in Wound Management edited by David Gray

Essential Wound Management: An introduction for undergraduates edited by David Gray, Richard White and Pam Cooper

Wound Healing: A systematic approach to advanced wound healing and management edited by David Gray, Richard White and Pam Cooper

Wounds UK — The Directory, 2006 edited by Richard White

Honey: A modern wound management product

edited by

Richard White, Rose Cooper, and Peter Molan

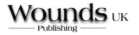

Wounds UK
Publishing

Advancis
Medical

Sponsored by:
Advancis Medical
Lowmoor Business Park
Kirkby-in-Ashfield
Nottingham
NG17 7JZ
United Kingdom
Tel: +44 (0)1623 751500
Fax: +44 (0)1623 757636
Email: enquiries@advancis.co.uk
Web: www.advancis.co.uk

Wounds UK Publishing, Wounds UK Limited, Suite 3.1, 36 Upperkirkgate,
Aberdeen AB10 1BA

British Library Cataloguing-in-Publication Data
A catalogue record is available for this book

Printed in the UK by Cromwell Press, Trowbridge, Wiltshire

CONTENTS

LIST OF CONTRIBUTORS

Rose Cooper BSc, PhD, PGCE is Principal Lecturer in Microbiology, University of Wales Institute Cardiff, UK

Cheryl Dunford RGN, MSc, PGCE is Lecturer in Tissue Viability, School of Nursing and Midwifery, Southampton University, UK

Ken Jones MPhil, PhD is a Principal Lecturer, Reader in the Department of Applied Sciences, University of Wales Institute Cardiff, UK

Andrew Kingsley RGN, BSc (Nursing) is CNS Tissue Viability at Northern Devon Healthcare Trust, UK

Lee Martin MD, FRCS is Consultant Surgeon, Aintree Hospitals Trust, Longmoor Lane, Liverpool, UK

Peter Molan BSc, PhD is Professor of Biological Sciences and Director of the Honey Research Unit, University of Waikato, New Zealand

Keith Morris BSc, MSc, PhD is a Reader in the Department of Applied Sciences, University of Wales Institute Cardiff, UK

Val Robson BSc (Hons), RGN is Clinical Nurse Specialist, Leg Ulcer Care, Aintree Hospitals Trust, Longmoor Lane, Liverpool, UK

Claire Newlands B Tech is Quality Manager — Medical, Comvita Medical, Comvita, New Zealand

Jackie Stephen-Haynes RGN, DN, DipH, BSc, MSC, A.N.P, PG Dip R, PG Dip ED is Lecturer and Practitioner in Tissue Viability for Worcestershire Primary Care Trusts and University College Worcester, UK

Richard White PhD, is Senior Research Fellow, Department of Tissue Viability, Aberdeen Royal Infirmary, Scotland

Young Mee Yoon PhD is Technical Manager — Medical, Comvita Medical, Comvita, New Zealand

FOREWORD

Faced with serious and worsening clinical problems caused by bacteria resistant to commonly used antibiotics, microbiologists are energetically investigating alternative approaches. One of these is the use of honey. Although associated with health from the very earliest times, it has been studied scientifically only comparatively recently. Two contributors to *Honey: A modern wound management product,* have made particularly significant contributions to this new understanding. Rose Cooper and colleagues at the University of Wales Institute in Cardiff, UK, have, for example, studied twenty strains of *Burkholderia cepacia* that were resistant to several different antibiotics. They isolated the bacteria from cystic fibrosis patients who were opportunistically infected with this bacterium, and found that all of the strains were susceptible to honey (Cooper *et al*, 2000).

More recently, in collaboration with Peter Molan at the University of Waikato in New Zealand, they found that eighteen strains of methicillin-resistant *Staphylococcus aureus* (MRSA), and seven strains of vancomycin-sensitive *Enterococcus faecalis* were also sensitive to Manuka and pasture honey (Cooper *et al*, 2002). All of these organisms came from infected wounds, and represent categories of bacteria that are responsible for some of the most challenging problems faced by clinicians trying to deal with intractable wound infections.

This, and other work, highlight the considerable potential of using honey to decontaminate wounds colonised by antibiotic-resistant bacteria. The prospect is doubly appealing since honey, in contrast to certain other topical antimicrobial agents, does not adversely affect human tissues. It is also inexpensive — and unlikely to create selective conditions that facilitate the emergence of further resistant strains.

These developments make the appearance of this book especially timely. Its compass, however, is far wider, covering a range of significant advances in both understanding and exploiting the actions of honey on wounds. Incorporating several groups of case histories, the book describes not only the antimicrobial action of honey, but also its capacity to combat prolonged, inappropriate inflammation, and to promote healing and tissue regeneration. These properties are especially notable in the context of the management of chronic, intractable wounds. The contributors deal with both the underlying science of the modes of action of honey and its practical applications. Also included is an account of the criteria for medical grade honey, which is important since the introduction in 2003 of the first Medical Devices impregnated with honey.

Honey is not a magic potion or universal panacea. Moreover, as Andrew Kingsley points out, it does have certain 'downsides'. Yet, its potent activities, together with its conspicuous safeness, amply justify the medical interest it is now attracting. While some of the health claims made for honey in the past appear fanciful in light of today's knowledge, this book clearly establishes that in one area, at least, it seems destined to find a significant niche in routine medical practice.

Dr Bernard Dixon, OBE, DSc

March 2005

References

Cooper RA, Wigley P, Burton NF (2000) Susceptibility of multiresistant strains of *Burkholderia cepacia* to honey. *Lett Appl Microbiol* **31**: 20

Cooper RA, Molan PC, Harding KG (2002) The sensitivity to honey of Gram-positive cocci of clinical significance from wounds. *J Appl Microbiol* **93**: 857

Preface

A definition of faith:

Confident belief in the truth or value of an idea or concept that does not rest on logical proof or material evidence.

The concept of honey being used today for the management of wounds requires a leap of faith from many people to proceed beyond the misconception that this is a traditional remedy, with no basis in scientific fact or evidence. However, the quality and depth of evidence is rapidly increasing and numerous wound care practitioners now regard the subject of this book as both scientifically based, and an important addition to modern wound healing.

I believe that this text will help those who are still undecided to recognise the value of medical grade honey as a viable wound treatment therapy, and also prove a useful reference guide to others already using regulated Medical Device honey products.

Advancis Medical is proud to be associated with this book and the medical Manuka honey programme. We wish to thank the editors and authors for their contributions. We would also like to thank them, and numerous unnamed clinical and microbiological specialists, for their willingness to have the initial leap in faith to investigate and pioneer the re-adoption of medical grade honey into mainstream medical practice.

Chris Hill
Sales and Marketing Manager
Advancis Medical
March 2005

Chapter 1

Mode of action

Peter Molan

Introduction

Honey is a substance produced by bees to store as a sugar food source collected as nectar from flowers (and occasionally from the sap of plants). Since the earliest recorded times, humans have taken this honey for use, not only as a food product, but also as a medicine, especially for wound care (Zumla and Lulat, 1989). The bees concentrate the dilute sugar solutions they collect from the plants by evaporating off most of the water. (Honey is typically 17% water, 80% sugars.) They also add enzymes, so that as the honey ripens in the comb its composition changes and it becomes impossible for microbes to grow in it and spoil the stored food. One of these enzymes converts sucrose, the major sugar in nectar and sap, into a more soluble mixture of glucose and fructose. This makes the saturated or supersaturated solution of sugars that is stored as honey. (The difference in texture between liquid honey and solid or 'creamed' honey is due to fine crystals of solidified glucose being suspended in the saturated syrup.) The sugar molecules in solution bind up water molecules, thereby denying microbes the water that is essential for their survival. Another enzyme added is glucose oxidase. This converts some of the glucose to gluconic acid, making honey too acidic for microbes to grow (honey has a pH of about 3.5) and, as a by-product of this reaction, forms hydrogen peroxide. This is a sporicidal antiseptic that sterilises the honey that is sealed in the comb. (When subsequently extracted from the comb, honey can be contaminated with microbial spores as the enzyme that produces hydrogen peroxide is inactive at that time because there is insufficient free water. These can survive the acidity and high sugar content.) These factors, which ensure the preservation of honey in the comb, are also useful in suppressing microbial growth when honey is applied to a wound.

Additionally, there are 'herbal' factors present which may be of benefit in wound care. Being the concentrated juice from plants, honey contains the various nutrients and herbal chemicals that come from the plants, such as: amino acids, other organic acids, enzymes, vitamins, acetylcholine, flavonoids, carotenoids, polyphenols, minerals and a wide variety of organic chemicals in trace quantities. These are what give different honeys their characteristic colours, flavours and aromas. The colour of honey is also due to products of the Maillard reaction[1] and caramelisation of its sugars, hence it gets darker in colour as it ages. Some of the plant-derived chemicals have antioxidant properties and some are known to have antibacterial properties.

It is for topical treatment of infections that honey has been most widely used as a medicine throughout history, and now that its use as a wound dressing has been 'rediscovered' by the medical profession, it is on infected wounds that it is mostly being used. The clinical definition of infection is that the area of the wound is showing the classical signs of inflammation (redness, swelling and pain). The clinical focus in treating wounds is to remove the cause of the inflammation by killing the infecting bacteria and removing any pus or dead tissue that provide a medium for their growth. Inflammation in a wound causes many problems, such as making the wound uncomfortable and difficult to manage, but the major problem is that it prevents the tissue repair processes from healing the wound. The various bioactivities of honey work through all of these facets to give rapid healing — honey rapidly debrides wounds (ie. cleans the wound by releasing pus or dead tissue), kills bacteria, directly suppresses inflammation, and stimulates the growth of the various types of cells involved in the production of new tissue to repair the wound.

The scourge of excessive inflammation

Inflammation is a vital part of the normal response to infection or injury, and is what starts the healing process. It normally lasts for one day but, if it is prolonged or if the inflammatory response is excessive in intensity, it can prevent healing or even cause further damage to tissues. Prolonged inflammation, at a level below that which causes damage, is the cause

---

1. Maillard reaction: one of a group of non-enzymatic reactions in which sugars react with amino acids, peptides or proteins to produce a brown colour in honey.

of fibrosis, seen as hypertrophic scarring in wounds. Inflammation in wounds also causes discomfort for patients and problems in dressing the wounds, because of the large amounts of exudate associated with it.

The prostaglandins are part of the inflammatory response. They give rise to pain and cause small arteries to open, increasing blood pressure locally and giving rise to oedema in the area of the wound, and exudation of plasma from the wound. Suppression of inflammation, as well as reduction of pain, reduces the oedema and exudate. The pressure building up in tissues from oedema can slow the healing process, as it restricts the flow of blood through the capillaries (Chant, 1999), thus starving the tissues of the oxygen and nutrients that are vital for leukocytes to fight infection and for fibroblasts to multiply for wound healing. The swelling also increases the distance for diffusion of oxygen and nutrients from the capillaries to the cells (Sinclair and Ryan, 1994).

The inflammatory response is initiated by the reaction of leukocytes when in contact with substances from bacterial cells, or to tissue factors released when there is physical damage. (In the case of burn injuries, there are large quantities of these tissue factors released, which accounts for the severe inflammation associated with burns.) Phagocytes that are activated as part of the initial inflammatory response produce hydrogen peroxide to destroy the bacteria and debris that they engulf. Some of this hydrogen peroxide leaks out of the cells, which serves to give a feed-back amplification of the inflammatory response, as the hydrogen peroxide attracts and stimulates other leucocytes to proliferate (Flohé et al, 1985). If this continues unchecked, the feed-back amplification can result in a vicious cycle that gives excessive levels of inflammation. Hydrogen peroxide was once widely used as an antiseptic, but has gone out of favour because it causes this inflammation. Although the hydrogen peroxide produced in honey may have the potential to cause inflammation, it is produced at very low levels, equivalent to about one thousandth of that in the 3% solution of hydrogen peroxide used as an antiseptic (Bang et al, 2003). However, there is also protection via the anti-inflammatory properties of honey (see below).

The hydrogen peroxide released by phagocytes can also be converted to reactive oxygen species (free radicals) in the tissues (Flohé et al, 1985). These free radicals are very reactive and can break down proteins, nucleic acids and cell membrane lipids, thus damaging or destroying tissue. Far greater damage to tissues results from the activation of proteases in the wound tissues by reactive oxygen species (Weiss et al, 1985; Ossanna et al, 1986; Peppin and Weiss, 1986). These protein-digesting enzymes are normally present in an inactive form (in the case of the matrix

3

metalloproteases), or are kept inactive by the presence of an inhibitor (in the case of the neutrophil serine protease). But, once activated, can destroy wound tissue. Thus, a wound can become ulcerated and a partial-thickness burn can become full-thickness. These activated proteases also have the potential to destroy the tissue growth factors which, being proteins, are essential for activation of the repair process.

In the case of reperfusion injury, hydrogen peroxide produced by a biochemical process is the initiator of the inflammatory response and the ongoing vicious cycle. When tissues are deprived of oxygen through obstruction of circulation, production of xanthine and alteration of the enzyme xanthine dehydrogenase to catalyse an oxidase type of reaction occurs. When the circulation is subsequently restored and the tissue is reperfused, the oxygen now available is used by the enzyme to oxidise xanthine, setting up production of hydrogen peroxide and reactive oxygen species (Bostek, 1989). This mechanism of initiation accounts for the inflammation in pressure ulcers (where circulation is cut off by pressure on the tissues then restored by relief of the pressure), and in varicose ulcers (where circulation is restricted by venous stasis then restored by elevating the legs), with the subsequent activation of proteases by the inflammatory reaction contributing to ulceration of the tissue.

Where the inflammation is less severe and insufficient to give erosion of tissue by activation of wound proteases, it can give excessive activation of fibroblasts, causing fibrosis, hypertrophic scarring and contractures. (Fibroblasts are the precursors of muscle cells, and use the same contractile fibres as muscle cells to pull the edges of a wound together. They also produce collagen fibres which form scar tissue.)

Although excessive or prolonged inflammation is a major problem in wounds, pharmaceutical anti-inflammatory substances are not generally used in wound treatment because they can impair healing through adverse effects on proliferating cells. Honey, however, has a potent anti-inflammatory action that not only has no adverse effects on the growth of cells, but actually gives a positive stimulation of their growth.

The anti-inflammatory properties of honey

Many clinical observations have been reported of reduced symptoms of inflammation when honey is applied to wounds (Burlando, 1978; Dumronglert, 1983; Efem, 1993; Hejase *et al*, 1996; Subrahmanyam,

1996; Subrahmanyam, 1998), and of it having a soothing effect when applied to wounds (Burlando, 1978; Keast-Butler, 1980; Subrahmanyam, 1993) and burns (Burlando, 1978; Subrahmanyam, 1993). The (reported) reduction of exudate in wounds dressed with honey is a great help when managing inflamed wounds (Burlando, 1978; Efem, 1993; Hejase et al, 1996; Al-Waili and Saloom, 1999; Betts and Molan, 2001; Alcaraz and Kelly, 2002; Ahmed et al, 2003). The anti-inflammatory action of honey is also seen in the reports of reducing scarring (Subrahmanyam, 1991; Efem, 1993; Subrahmanyam, 1994; Al-Waili and Saloom, 1999; Dunford et al, 2000a, b) and contractures (Subrahmanyam et al, 2001). As well as these clinical observations, it has been demonstrated in animal models that honey gives reduced inflammation compared with various controls; histological studies finding reduced numbers of inflammatory cells present in deep (Postmes et al, 1997) and superficial (Burlando, 1978) burns and in full-thickness wounds (Gupta et al, 1992; Kumar et al, 1993; Oryan and Zaker, 1998). These effects are due to components other than the sugar in honey (Burlando, 1978; Postmes et al, 1997). Similar evidence has also come from a study of biopsy samples from burn wound tissue of hospital patients (Subrahmanyam, 1998). The anti-inflammatory action of honey is not just a consequence of removing the stimulus for inflammation by clearing infection and debriding the wound, as has been observed in experimental wounds in which there were few or no bacteria present (Burlando, 1978; Kandil et al, 1987; El-Banby et al, 1989; Gupta et al, 1992; Kumar et al, 1993; Postmes et al, 1997; Oryan and Zaker, 1998). There has also been a direct demonstration of the anti-inflammatory properties of honey in a standard test for anti-inflammatory agents, where it decreased the stiffness of inflamed wrist joints of guinea pigs (Church, 1954). It has also been reported that, when given orally, honey lowers plasma prostaglandin concentrations in normal individuals (Al-Waili and Boni, 2003).

The component of honey responsible for its anti-inflammatory activity has not been identified, but it may be due to the antioxidant activity of honey. There are significant levels of antioxidants in honey (Frankel et al, 1998; Gheldof and Engeseth, 2002; Gheldof et al, 2002; Gheldof et al, 2003; Schramm et al, 2003), including some which complex with iron to stop it catalysing the Fenton reaction[2]. This reaction forms free radicals from hydrogen peroxide (Buntting,

---

2. Fenton reaction: the formation of free radicals from the non-enzymatic reaction of iron (Fe^{2+}) with hydrogen peroxide (H_2O_2); a reaction of importance in the oxidative stress in blood cells and various tissues.

2001); these free radicals serve to recruit more leukocytes into areas of inflammation, as a self-amplification of the inflammatory response (Flohé *et al*, 1985). The mechanism of this self-amplification of the inflammatory response is oxidative activation of the nuclear transcription factor NF-κB, which then promotes the production of pro-inflammatory cytokines by leukocytes (Grimble, 1994) and stimulate the activity of the fibroblasts, thus giving hypergranulation and fibrosis (Murrell *et al*, 1990). It is the free radicals formed from hydrogen peroxide, rather than hydrogen peroxide itself, that are responsible for the activation of the transcription factor NF-κB (Schreck *et al*, 1991), and this activation can be prevented by antioxidants (Grimble, 1994). A study carried out on burn wounds has shown that application of antioxidants to mop up free radicals reduces inflammation (Tanaka *et al*, 1995). In a clinical trial it was found that honey dressings prevented partial-thickness burns from converting to full-thickness burns which would have needed plastic surgery (Subrahmanyam, 1998).

Clearance of infection

Applying honey dressings to wounds has been reported to:

- clear infection rapidly (Cavanagh *et al*, 1970; Armon, 1980; Braniki, 1981; Phuapradit and Saropala, 1992; Efem, 1993; Anoukoum *et al*, 1998; Robson *et al*, 2000; Betts and Molan, 2001; Kingsley, 2001; Subrahmanyam *et al*, 2001; Alcaraz and Kelly, 2002)
- heal deeply infected surgical wounds (Cavanagh *et al*, 1970; Armon, 1980; Bergman *et al*, 1983; McInerney, 1990; Phuapradit and Saropala, 1992; Vardi *et al*, 1998; Al-Waili and Saloom, 1999; Cooper *et al*, 2001)
- halt advancing necrotising fasciitis (Efem, 1993; Hejase *et al*, 1996).

Wounds not responding to conventional therapy with antibiotics and antiseptics have been healed by application of honey dressings (Efem, 1993; Harris, 1994; Wood *et al*, 1997; Vardi *et al*, 1998; Dunford *et al*, 2000a, b; Cooper *et al*, 2001), including wounds infected with methicillin-resistant *Staphylococcus aureus* (MRSA) (Dunford *et al*, 2000a; Natarajan *et al*, 2001), *Pseudomonas aeruginosa* (Dunford *et al*, 2000b) and other bacteria resistant to antibiotics (Al-Waili and Saloom, 1999).

The laboratory evidence for the potent broad-spectrum antimicrobial activity of honey is covered in *Chapter 2*, as is the stimulatory action of honey on leukocytes — another mechanism by which honey may work to clear infection from wounds. There is no clear evidence of the ability of the antibacterial activity of honey to diffuse down into wound tissue when applied as a wound dressing. But, the suppression by honey of growth of any bacteria already present on the surface of the wound means that there is not the problem of malodorous dressings when hydrocolloid dressings are used. Being a source of toxins and pyrogens, honey also removes the problem of bacteria growing on the wound surface. However, the rapid clearance of a deep-seated infection (Cooper *et al*, 2001) and of boils with unbroken skin (Betts and Molan, 2002) by topical application of honey indicates that the antibacterial activity of honey probably does diffuse though skin. If this is so, it is important to use a honey with a high level of antibacterial activity (*Chapter 2*) to achieve an effective level of antibacterial activity below the surface. When diffusion occurs, there is a gradient formed of decreasing concentration from the source (in this case, the dressing on the surface of the wound). As illustrated in *Figure 1.1*, the minimum concentration of antibacterial component that will stop bacterial growth will be deeper down in the wound tissue if the source has a higher concentration. It is also important to keep a substantial quantity of honey on the surface (eg. by using a dressing pad soaked with honey), so that the concentration of antibacterial activity on the surface does not become low through dilution by exudate, or depletion by diffusion into the underlying tissue

Deodorising action

Honey rapidly deodorises wounds (McInerney, 1990; Subrahmanyam, 1991; Phuapradit and Saropala, 1992; Efem, 1993; Subrahmanyam, 1993; Hejase *et al*, 1996; Subrahmanyam, 1996; Dunford *et al*, 2000a, b; Kingsley, 2001; Alcaraz and Kelly, 2002; Stewart, 2002; Ahmed *et al*, 2003). On fungating (malignant) wounds where no other treatment could control the malodour, dressing the wound with honey was found to remove the malodour within twenty-four hours (Julie Betts, Waikato Hospital: personal communication). Honey is now being used routinely at Waikato Hospital on fungating wounds, not only for odour control, but also because it reduces the inflammation and level of exudate that is a common problem with this type of wound.

The rapid deodorising of wounds from honey dressings is probably due to more than just antibacterial action. The malodorous substances that bacteria produce in wounds, such as, ammonia, amines and sulphur compounds, are formed from the metabolism of amino acids derived from decomposed serum and tissue proteins. Bacteria metabolise glucose in preference to amino acids, thus, in the presence of honey (composition of 30%–40%), the malododorous compounds are not formed (Nychas *et al*, 1988).

Barrier function

The high viscosity of honey provides a physical barrier to infection of wounds from external contamination, the effectiveness of which is increased by the antibacterial activity of the honey (as long as the honey used is selected to have good antibacterial activity). This feature is particularly useful where it is preferable to avoid occluding highly exudative wounds, such as burn wounds, and thus encourage growth of bacteria, particularly *Pseudomonas spp*, in the moist conditions created. Prophylactic use of honey dressings has been found to solve a problem of skin grafts frequently becoming infected with *Pseudomonas spp* (Robson, 2000). This raises the suggestion of using honey dressings routinely on surgical wounds to protect at-risk patients from acquiring nosocomial infection with MRSA — the demonstrated sensitivity of MRSA to honey (*Chapter 2*) and the reports of honey dressings healing wounds already infected with MRSA (Dunford *et al*, 2000a; Natarajan *et al*, 2001) indicate that it is likely to be effective as a prophylactic treatment. It is also likely to be effective as a prophylactic treatment for the other major route of nosocomial infection with MRSA, ie. sites where medical devices penetrate the skin, as indicated by the favourable results reported from a trial conducted on central vein catheter exit sites (Mutjaba Quadri, 1999).

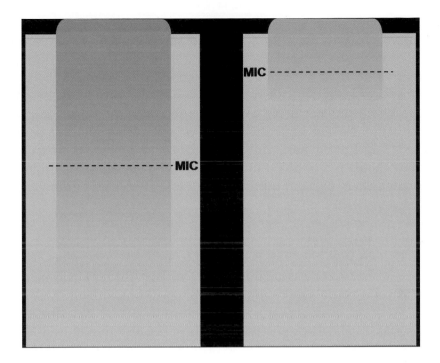

Figure 1.1: Illustration of concentration gradients set up by diffusion into underlying tissue of antibacterial activity of honey from high-activity and low-activity honey on the surface of the skin. 'MIC' shows the position on the gradients of the minimum inhibitory concentration of the antibacterial activity (ie. the minimum concentration that will stop bacterial growth). Thus, the functional components of a high activity honey will diffuse deeper into the tissues and have a greater range of antibacterial activity

Provision of the optimum moist healing environment

Honey dressings on wounds provide a moist healing environment: a feature sought in most modern wound dressings to obtain conditions necessary for optimum growth of the cells involved in the repair process. But, unlike other dressings, honey does this without the associated problems of encouraging microbial growth and maceration of surrounding skin that can result from the moist conditions. The antibacterial activity of honey prevents bacterial growth without any cytotoxic effects which could otherwise slow healing; and the osmotic action of its high sugar content will tend to draw fluid out from skin rather then let it soak in, even if honey gets diluted by large amounts of exudate. This means that there is no need to trim honey dressings to the shape of the wound bed or to use protective coverings on peri-wound skin, and there is no restriction on using occlusive secondary dressings. It has been suggested that the osmotic effect would dehydrate wound tissues but, in a paper on the use of sugar as a wound dressing, it has been pointed out that where there is a circulation of blood underneath to replace fluid lost from cells, the osmotic effect of sugar on the surface just creates an outflow of fluid (Chirife *et al*, 1982).

Also, unlike other dressings, honey dressings are easy to remove (Blomfield, 1973; Wadi *et al*, 1987; Farouk *et al*, 1988; Dunford *et al*, 2000a, b; Robson *et al*, 2000; Betts and Molan, 2001; Cooper *et al*, 2001; Alcaraz and Kelly, 2002; Richards, 2002; Stewart, 2002; Misirlioglu *et al*, 2003), causing no pain on changing dressings (Bulman, 1955; McInerney, 1990; Weheida *et al*, 1991; Subrahmanyam, 1993; Subrahmanyam, 1998; Dunford and Hanano, 2004). This is because the outflow of fluid from the wound bed created by the osmotic action of the honey forms a layer of diluted honey in contact with the wound bed. This fluid interface allows the dressings to be lifted off painlessly, preventing the tearing away of newly regenerated tissue which can happen when an adherent wound dressing is pulled off.

Debriding action

There are many reports that wounds dressed with honey are rapidly debrided to give a clean granulating wound bed (Cavanagh *et al*, 1970; Armon, 1980; Braniki, 1981; Efem, 1993; Subrahmanyam, 1998; Dunford *et al*, 2000b; Alcaraz and Kelly, 2002; Ahmed *et al*, 2003), slough and necrotic tissue painlessly lifting off (Subrahmanyam, 1991; Efem, 1993; Subrahmanyam, 1993; Hejase *et al*, 1996; Subrahmanyam, 1996). Although induction of autolytic debridement is a feature of all wound dressings that give a moist environment, the debriding action of honey is faster than with other dressings and, on sloughy wounds, is about as rapid as that experienced using maggots (Julie Betts, Waikato Hospital: personal communication). Where there is hard eschar, maggot therapy provides a faster method of debridement as the maggots appear to burrow under the edges of the eschar, but honey dressings will remove hard eschar, especially if this is scored to aid penetration of the honey, and if the honey is diluted with water or saline so that it softens the eschar. Furthermore, using honey instead of maggots, removes the problems of obtaining a supply of freshly prepared material, of ensuring that the wound is not too wet (causing drowning) or too dry (killing by dehydration), or of keeping the maggots in place, and of overcoming patients' unease with the squirming movement of the maggots.

The debriding action of maggots is due to the proteolytic enzyme activity they secrete, but with honey there does not appear to be a direct proteolytic activity involved: the existence of protein-digesting enzyme activity in honey has not been reported. Therefore, there must be a mechanism by which honey activates dormant proteolytic enzyme activity within the wound tissue, but in a controlled way so as not to cause unwanted digestion of the tissue. There is a strong association between high protease activity and impaired wound healing, and dressings are now being produced that inhibit or bind up and inactivate excessive protease activity in wounds that would otherwise be digesting wound tissue (Edwards _et al_, 2001; Cullen _et al_, 2002; Edwards _et al_, 2004). As mentioned earlier, the tissue-digesting collagenase and elastase enzyme activity in wounds is activated by oxidation. The antioxidant activity of honey can be expected to suppress this, just as the anti-inflammatory activity suppresses the infiltration of elastase-secreting neutrophils. This decreases the amount of enzyme released and, subsequently, the activity of that enzyme. The most likely explanation of the debriding activity induced by honey is that it promotes conversion of inactive plasminogen in the wound matrix to the active form, plasmin. This is an enzyme that functions to break down fibrin clots which attach slough and eschar to the wound bed. This action of honey could also be attributed to its anti-inflammatory activity, as inflammation causes inhibition of fibrinolysis by elevating the level of PAI-1 (plasminogen activator inhibitor 1) and thus preventing plasminogen from being converted to the active enzyme plasmin (Esmon, 2004). Fibrin is very common in chronic wounds (Schultz _et al_, 2003). (The enzyme streptokinase that is often used to debride wounds functions by activating plasminogen.)

The osmotic action of honey may also assist, as drawing out lymph from the wound tissues gives a constantly replenished supply of plasminogen at the interface of the wound bed and the overlying slough. Another advantage of this osmotic action of honey is that it washes the surface of the wound bed from beneath. This would account for the long-known feature of honey dressings to remove dirt with the dressing (Zaiß, 1934), making such dressings an excellent way of cleaning up grazes in which grit has become embedded.

Stimulation of healing

Wounds dressed with honey often have a rapid rate of healing. Honey is also able to start the healing process in dormant wounds. Honey has been reported to promote the formation of granulation tissue and to stimulate the growth of epithelium over wounds. Clinical evidence of the use of honey on wounds is reviewed in *Chapter 9*. It has also been reported that honey is a reliable alternative to conventional dressing for the management of skin excoriation around stomas (ileostomy and colostomy), giving a more rapid epithelialisation of the raw surface (Aminu *et al*, 2000). These clinical observations of the stimulatory effect of honey on tissue growth in wounds have been confirmed by measurements and histological observations in studies of experimental wounds in animals (Burlando, 1978; Bergman *et al*, 1983; Gupta *et al*, 1992; Kumar *et al*, 1993; Suguna *et al*, 1993; Postmes *et al*, 1997), where honey treatment has been shown to give statistically significant improvements. In these experimental wounds, honey has also been shown to stimulate the synthesis of collagen (Suguna *et al*, 1992) and other connective tissue components (Suguna *et al*, 1993), and to stimulate angiogenesis (development of new blood vessels) (Gupta *et al*, 1992; Kumar *et al*, 1993).

Stimulation of angiogenesis is an important feature for promotion of healing, as the supply of oxygen is the rate-limiting factor in tissue repair (Silver, 1980), granulation tissue being granules of fibroblasts growing where new capillary beds form. The anti-inflammatory activity of honey would also assist by decreasing oedema and, consequently, the pressure on capillaries which restricts blood flow and the supply of oxygen to the regenerating wound tissues. The acidity of honey would also help with oxygenation, as acidification of wounds speeds the rate of healing by increasing the release of oxygen from haemoglobin (Kaufman *et al*, 1985). The newly-formed capillaries supply essential nutrients to growing fibroblasts, another factor limiting the rate of healing — it has been demonstrated that wounds heal faster if a nutrient mixture is applied topically (Viljanto and Raekallio, 1976; Niinikoski *et al*,

1977; Silvetti, 1981; Kaufman *et al*, 1984). There is a wide range of minerals, including the trace elements of nutrition, and of amino acids and vitamins contained in honey (Haydak *et al*, 1975; White, 1975). Although these are present in amounts too low to be of nutritional significance when compared with the recommended daily intake, they are, on average, present at levels like those circulating in the blood. This topical supply of nutrients would be augmented by the osmotic action of honey drawing lymph from the underlying capillaries, thus creating a constant flow of nutrients for cells which may be somewhat distant from the functioning capillaries deeper down. Another way in which honey may promote healing is by supplying glucose to the epithelial cells, as these have to build up an internal store of carbohydrate to provide the energy they need to migrate across the surface of a wound to restore skin cover (Silver, 1980). The level of glucose in the wound fluid of chronic wounds is very low (Schultz *et al*, 2003). The sugars in honey would also provide an energy source for the macrophages working in the wound, as glycolysis is their major mechanism for energy production, and is dependent on a supply of glucose or fructose. Glycolysis is the only means of cells obtaining energy in the absence of oxygen, so the supply of sugars from honey would allow them to function in damaged tissues where the oxygen supply is often poor (Ryan and Majno, 1977).

Another possible way that honey may work to stimulate wound repair is through its production of hydrogen peroxide, as hydrogen peroxide activates the insulin receptor complexes on cells (Czech *et al*, 1974; Helm and Gunn, 1986; Koshio *et al*, 1988). Activation triggers a chain of molecular events in the cell that stimulates the uptake of glucose and amino acids, and promotes anabolic metabolism, giving cell growth. Topical or intravenous application of insulin to wounds, stimulates the rate of wound healing (Lopez and Mena, 1968; Belfield *et al*, 1970; Pierre *et al*, 1998). By this mechanism, honey may stimulate the uptake and anabolic metabolism of the nutrients it supplies to wound tissues.

The stimulation of angiogenesis by honey, that has been observed experimentally when honey is applied to wounds, could also be via its production of hydrogen peroxide, as topical application of hydrogen peroxide has been found to enhance cutaneous blood recruitment in ischaemic ulcers (Tur *et al*, 1995). In vascular, smooth muscle cells, hydrogen peroxide is endogenously produced as part of the process of response to stimulation by platelet-derived growth factor, and exogenous hydrogen peroxide in the concentration range of 0.1 to 1.0 mmol/l will also function in the response (Rao and Berk, 1992). The promotion of formation of granulation tissue by honey may also be via the stimulation of growth of fibroblasts by the hydrogen peroxide produced in honey, as hydrogen peroxide has been found to stimulate the proliferation of fibroblasts (Chung *et al*, 1993). There is a large amount of evidence that hydrogen peroxide is involved in many cell types in the body as a stimulus for cell multiplication, by acting at various points in the mechanisms of the cells that control the cycle of cell growth and division (Burdon, 1995). It has been proposed that low concentrations of hydrogen peroxide might be used to stimulate wound healing in place of the expensive cell growth factors used for this purpose (Burdon, 1995; Postmes and Vandeputte, 1999). However, this is feasible only if the concentration could be carefully controlled to avoid tissue damage (Chung *et al*, 1993). This is possible with the controlled sustained release of hydrogen peroxide that occurs in honey.

Another possibility is that the stimulation of tissue repair is a down-stream effect of the stimulation by honey of cytokine production by leukocytes. The production of cytokines, as part of the initial inflammatory response, normally starts off the healing process. There is good evidence for the ability of honey in quite dilute solution to stimulate such a response in leukocytes in cell culture. This is discussed in *Chapter 2*.

Safety in use

Honey is extremely safe to use. In the 500-plus cases reported in publications on using honey on wounds, and the 140-plus cases reported of using honey in ophthalmology, there has been no mention of any adverse effects. A large number of other cases that have not been published are known to the author and, again, there have been no adverse effects observed in any of these, with the exception of one case where there appeared to be an allergic reaction on the skin around the wound. With honey, there are no reported cytotoxic effects that would slow the healing process, whereas all antiseptics in common use can be harmful to body tissues (Tatnall *et al*, 1991), including silver as released from nanocrystalline silver dressings (Poon and Burd, 2004).

There have been reports of honey causing a stinging pain when applied to wounds (Dunford *et al*, 2000b; Robson *et al*, 2001; Ahmed *et al*, 2003). This appears to be due to the acidity of honey, as pain is not experienced when neutralised honey is used (Dunford *et al*, 2000b;

Betts and Molan, 2001). The pain experienced does not seem to be indicative of damage being done to the wound, as wounds have healed rapidly in cases where patients have endured the pain to benefit from the stimulation of healing that they see, and in cases where analgesia has been used (personal communications from numerous clinicians). There is evidence that honey stimulates nocioceptors (Al-Swayeh and Ali, 1998), nerve endings that create a pain sensation in response to heat, acidity and some organic chemicals such as those in ginger and chilli. It is of interest that patients have been reported to experience a 'peppery' sensation from application of honey to their ulcers (Oluwatosin _et al_, 2000). It may be that it is not a direct effect of the acidity of honey, as neutralising honey could affect the ionisation of some of its components and make them unable to fit in the nocioceptors. It is possible that in some patients these nerve endings are sensitised and are more responsive to the acidity and/or the component organic chemicals of honey.

However, there are many reports of honey relieving pain (Al-Waili and Saloom, 1999; Dunford _et al_, 2000a, b; Cooper _et al_, 2001; Subrahmanyam _et al_, 2001; Richards, 2002; Stewart, 2002; Misirlioglu _et al_, 2003). In a trial in which pain was measured on a visual analogue scale, the pain experienced with a honey-soaked gauze dressing was found to be one-third less than with saline-soaked gauze and paraffin gauze, but slightly more than with a hydrocolloid dressing (Misirlioglu _et al_, 2003). In another trial, where the comfort of honey dressings on chronic venous leg ulcers was investigated, six patients experienced a transient stinging pain, and eight experienced a lasting pain, but only some of the times the dressing was applied (Dunford and Hanano, 2004). However, in this trial, the overall result was that pain was significantly reduced by the honey dressings, and the patient satisfaction with the honey dressings was high.

Other cases where honey is reported to cause pain are few. In one of these, there was pain experienced by the patient for the first twenty to thirty minutes (Dunford _et al_, 2000b). In another case, a patient experienced moderate pain for fifteen to thirty minutes after honey was applied (Robson _et al_, 2001). In a clinical trial of honey dressings, one of the sixty patients treated with honey withdrew because the dressings caused pain (Ahmed _et al_, 2003). In a pilot trial in which the author participated (Betts and Molan, 2002), six of the twenty patients recruited withdrew because of the pain caused by honey on the wound. This probably reflects the recruitment criterion of infected or heavily colonised wounds for the trial, as it was observed that pain was experienced only in inflamed wounds. Patients who found honey very painful when their wounds were inflamed experienced no problem with pain once the inflammation had subsided. Similarly, in the trial where the comfort of honey dressings on chronic venous leg ulcers was investigated, the six patients who withdrew from the trial because of the honey being painful (out of a total of forty participants), had a higher than average pain level before the start of the honey dressings (Dunford and Hanano, 2004).

Conclusion

The concerted action of the various physical properties and bioactivities in honey explains the remarkable results obtained clinically, especially when appropriately selected honeys are used and sufficient honey is held in place on the wound for these factors to work. Although some of the mechanisms of action are speculative, there is, nevertheless, a great deal of published evidence for honey having such actions on wounds. The excellent clinical evidence of overall effectiveness is presented in *Chapter 9*. The use of honey on human beings over a period of more than 4,000 years, with no adverse effects coming to light, is evidence of its effectiveness as a healing agent.

References

Ahmed AK, Hoekstra MJ, Hage JJ, Karim RB (2003) Honey-medicated dressing: transformation of an ancient remedy into modern therapy. *Ann Plast Surg* **50**(2): 143–7; discussion 147–8

Alcaraz A, Kelly J (2002). Treatment of an infected venous leg ulcer with honey dressings. *Br J Nurs* **11**(13): 859–60, 862, 864–6

Al-Swayeh OA, Ali ATM (1998) Effect of ablation of capsaicin-sensitive neurons on gastric protection by honey and sucralfate. *Hepato-Gastroenterology* **45**(19): 297–302

Al-Waili NS, Boni NS (2003) Natural honey lowers plasma prostaglandin concentrations in normal individuals. *J Medicinal Food* **6**(2): 129–33

Al-Waili NS, Saloom KY (1999) Effects of topical honey on post-operative wound infections due to gram positive and gram negative bacteria following caesarean sections and hysterectomies. *Eur J Med Res* **4**: 126–30

Aminu SR, Hassan AW, Babayo UD (2000) Another use of honey. _Trop Doct_ **30**: 250–51

Anoukoum T, Attipou KK, Ayite A, James YE, James K (1998) Le traitment des gangrenes perineales et de la sphere genitale par du miel. _Tunis Med_ **76**(5): 132–5

Armon PJ (1980) The use of honey in the treatment of infected wounds. _Trop Doct_ **10**: 91

Bang LM, Buntting C, Molan PC (2003) The effect of dilution on the rate of hydrogen peroxide production in honey and its implications for wound healing. _J Alternative Complementary Med_ **9**(2): 267–73

Belfield WO, Golinsky S, Compton MD (1970) The use of insulin in open wound healing. _Vet Med: Small Animal Clinician_ **65**(5): 455–60

Bergman A, Yanai J, Weiss J, Bell D, David MP (1983) Acceleration of wound healing by topical application of honey. An animal model. _Am J Surg_ **145**: 374–6

Betts JA, Molan PC (2001) A pilot trial of honey as a wound dressing has shown the importance of the way that honey is applied to wounds. 11th Conference of the European Wound Management Association, Dublin, Ireland

Betts JA, Molan PC (2002) Results of a pilot trial of manuka honey as a dressing for infected chronic wounds. 4th Australian Wound Management Association Conference, Adelaide, Australia

Blomfield R (1973) Honey for decubitus ulcers. _J Am Med Assoc_ **224**(6): 905

Bloomfield E (1976) Old remedies. _J R Coll Gen Pract_ **26**: 576

Bostek CC (1989) Oxygen toxicity: An introduction. _J Am Assoc Nurse Anesthetists_ **57**(3): 231–7

Braniki FJ (1981) Surgery in Western Kenya. _Ann R Coll Surg Engl_ **63**: 348–52

Bulman MW (1955) Honey as a surgical dressing. _Middlesex Hospital J_ **55**: 188–9

Buntting C (2001) _The production of hydrogen peroxide by honey and its relevance to wound healing._ University of Waikato, New Zealand

Burdon RH (1995) Superoxide and hydrogen peroxide in relation to mammalian cell proliferation. _Free Radic Biol Med_ **18**(4): 775–94

Burlando F (1978) Sull'azione terapeutica del miele nelle ustioni. _Minerva Dermatologica_ **113**: 699–706

Cavanagh D, Beazley J, Ostapowicz F (1970) Radical operation for carcinoma of the vulva. A new approach to wound healing. _J Obstet Gynaecol British Commonwealth_ **77**(11): 1037–40

Chant A (1999) The biomechanics of leg ulceration. _Ann R Coll Surg Engl_ **81**: 80–5

Chirife J, Scarmato G, Herszage L (1982) Scientific basis for use of granulated sugar in treatment of infected wounds. *Lancet* **i** (6 March): 560–1

Chung LY, Schmidt RJ, Andrews AM, Turner TD (1993) A study of hydrogen peroxide generation by, and antioxidant activity of, Granuflex™ (DuoDERM™) Hydrocolloid Granules and some other hydrogel/hydrocolloid wound management materials. *Br J Dermatol* **129**(2): 145–53

Church J (1954) Honey as a source of the anti-stiffness factor. *Federation Proc Am Physiol Soc* **13**(1): 26

Cooper RA, Molan PC, Krishnamoorthy L, Harding KG (2001) Manuka honey used to heal a recalcitrant surgical wound. *Eur J Clin Microbiol Infect Dis* **20**: 758–9

Cullen B, Smith R, McCulloch E, Silcock D, Morrison L (2002) Mechanism of action of PROMOGRAN, a protease modulating matrix, for the treatment of diabetic foot ulcers. *Wound Repair Regen* **10**(1): 16–25

Czech MP, Lawrence Jr, JC, Lynn WS (1974) Evidence for the involvement of sulphydryl oxidation in the regulation of fat cell hexose transport by insulin. *Proc Natl Acad Sci U S A* **71**(10): 4173–77

Dumronglert E (1983) A follow-up study of chronic wound healing dressing with pure natural honey. *J Natl Res Council Thailand* **15**(2): 39–66

Dunford C, Cooper R, Molan PC (2000a) Using honey as a dressing for infected skin lesions. *Nurs Times* **96**(14 NT-plus): 7–9

Dunford C, Cooper R, Molan PC, White R (2000) The use of honey in wound management. *Nurs Standard* **15**(11): 63–8

Dunford CE, Hanano R (2004) Acceptability to patients of a honey dressing for non-healing venous leg ulcers. *J Wound Care* **13**(5): 193–7

Edwards JV, Howley P, Cohen IK (2004) In vitro inhibition of human neutrophil elastase by oleic acid albumin formulations from derivatized cotton wound dressings. *Int J Pharm* **284**(1–2): 1–12

Edwards JV, Yager, DR, Cohen IK, Diegelmann RF, Montante S, Bertoniere N, Bopp AF (2001) Modified cotton gauze dressings that selectively absorb neutrophil elastase activity in solution. *Wound Repair Regen* **9**(1): 50–8

Efem SEE (1993) Recent advances in the management of Fournier's gangrene: Preliminary observations. *Surgery* **113**(2): 200–4

El-Banby M, Kandil A, Abou-Sehly G, El-Sherif ME, Abdel-Wahed K (1989) Healing effect of floral honey and honey from sugar-fed bees on surgical wounds (animal model). Fourth International Conference on Apiculture in Tropical Climates, Cairo, International Bee Research Association, London

Esmon CT (2004) Crosstalk between inflammation and thrombosis. *Maturitas* **47**(4): 305–14

Farouk A, Hassan T, Kashif H, Khalid SA, Mutawali I, Wadi M (1988) Studies on Sudanese bee honey: laboratory and clinical evaluation. *Int J Crude Drug Res* **26**(3): 161–8

Flohé L, Beckmann R, Giertz H, Loschen G (1985) Oxygen-centred free radicals as mediators of inflammation. In: Sies H, *Oxidative Stress*. Academic Press, London, Orlando: 403–35

Frankel S, Robinson GE, Berenbaum MR (1998) Antioxidant capacity and correlated characteristics of 14 unifloral honeys. *J Apicultural Res* **37**(1): 27–31

Gheldof N, Engeseth NJ (2002) Antioxidant capacity of honeys from various floral sources based on the determination of oxygen radical absorbance capacity and inhibition of in vitro lipoprotein oxidation in human serum samples. *J Agricultural Food Chemistry* **50**(10): 3050–55

Gheldof N, Wang X, Engeseth NJ (2002) Identification and quantification of antioxidant components of honeys from various floral sources. *J Agricultural Food Chemistry* **50**: 5870–77

Gheldof N, Wang XH, Engeseth NJ (2003) Buckwheat honey increases serum antioxidant capacity in humans. *J Agricultural Food Chemistry* **51**(5): 1500–5

Grimble GF (1994) Nutritional antioxidants and the modulation of inflammation: theory and practice. *New Horizons* **2**(2): 175–85

Gupta SK, Singh H, Varshney AC, Prakash P (1992) Therapeutic efficacy of honey in infected wounds in buffaloes. *Indian J Animal Sciences* **62**(6): 521–3

Harris S (1994) Honey for the treatment of superficial wounds: a case report and review. *Primary Intention* **2**(4): 18–23

Haydak MH, Crane E, Duisberg H, Gochnauer TA, Morse RA, White JW, Wix P (1975) *Biological Properties of Honey*. Heinemann, London

Hejase MJ, Bihrle R, Coogan CL (1996) Genital Fournier's gangrene: experience with 38 patients. *Urology* **47**(5): 734–9

Helm BA, Gunn JM (1986) The effect of insulinomimetic agents on protein degradation in H35 hepatoma cells. *Mol Cell Biochem* **71**(2): 159–66

Hutton DJ (1966) Treatment of pressure sores. *Nurs Times* **62**(46): 1533–34

Kandil A, El-Banby M, Abdel-Wahed K, Abou-Sehly G, Ezzat N (1987) Healing effect of true floral and false nonfloral honey on medical wounds. *J Drug Res* (Cairo) **17**(1–2): 71–5

Kaufman T, Eichenlaub EH, Angel MF, Levin M, Futrell JW (1985) Topical acidification promotes healing of experimental deep partial thickness skin burns: a randomised double-blind preliminary study. *Burns* **12**: 84–9

Kaufman T, Levin M, Hurwitz DJ (1984) The effect of topical hyperalimentation on wound healing rate and granulation tissue formation of experimental deep second degree burns in guinea-pigs. *Burns* **10**(4): 252–6

Keast-Butler J (1980) Honey for necrotic malignant breast ulcers. *Lancet* **ii** (11 October): 809

Kingsley A (2001) The use of honey in the treatment of infected wounds: case studies. *Br J Nurs* **10**(22) Tissue Viability Supplement: s13–s20

Koshio O, Akanuma Y, Kasuga M (1988) Hydrogen peroxide stimulates tyrosine phosphorylation of the insulin recepter and its tyrosine kinase activity in intact cells. *Biochem J* **250**: 95–101

Kumar A, Sharma, V K; Singh, H P; Prakash, P; Singh, S P (1993) Efficacy of some indigenous drugs in tissue repair in buffaloes. *Indian Veterinary J* **70**(1): 42–4

Lopez JE, Mena B (1968) Local insulin for diabetic gangrene. *Lancet* **i**: 1199

McInerney RJF (1990) Honey — a remedy rediscovered. *J R Soc Med* **83**: 127

Misirlioglu A, Eroglu S, Karacaoglan N, Akan M, Akoz T, Yildirim S (2003) Use of honey as an adjunct in the healing of split-thickness skin graft donor site. *Dermatol Surg* **29**(2): 168–72

Murrell, GAC, Francis MJO, Bromley L (1990) Modulation of fibroblast proliferation by oxygen free radicals. *Biochem J* **265**: 659–65

Mutjaba Quadri KH (1999) Manuka honey for central vein catheter exit site care. *Semin Dialysis* **12**(5): 397–8

Natarajan S, Williamson D, Grey J, Harding KG, Cooper RA (2001) Healing of an MRSA-colonised, hydroxyurea-induced leg ulcer with honey. *J Dermatol Treatment* **12**: 33–6

Niinikoski J, Kivisaari J, Viljanto J (1977) Local hyperalimentation of experimental granulation tissue. *Acta Chiropida Scand* **143**: 201–6

Nychas GJ, Dillon VM, Board RG (1988) Glucose, the key substrate in the microbiological changes in meat and certain meat products. *Biotechnol Appl Biochem* **10**: 203–31

Oluwatosin OM, Olabanji JK, Oluwatosin OA, Tijani LA, Onyechi HU (2000) A comparison of topical honey and phenytoin in the treatment of chronic leg ulcers. *Afri J Med Sci* **29**(1): 31–4

Oryan A, Zaker SR (1998) Effects of topical application of honey on cutaneous wound healing in rabbits. *J Veterinary Med* **Series A45** (3): 181–8

Ossanna PJ, Test ST, Matheson NR, Regiani S, Weiss SJ (1986) Oxidative regulation of neutrophil elastase-alpha-1-proteinase inhibitor interactions. *J Clinical Investigation* **77**: 1939–51

Peppin GJ, Weiss SJ (1986) Activation of the endogenous metalloproteinase, gelatinase, by triggered human neutrophils. *Proc Natl Acad Sci U S A* **83**: 4322–26

Phuapradit W, Saropala N (1992) Topical application of honey in treatment of abdominal wound disruption. *Aust N Z J Obstet Gynaecol* **32**(4): 381–4

Pierre EJ, Barrow RE, Hawkins HK, Nguyen TT, Sakurai Y, Desai M, Wolfe RR, Herndon DN (1998) Effects of insulin on wound healing. *J Trauma, Injury, Infect Crit Care* **44**(2): 342–5

Poon VK, Burd A (2004) In vitro cytotoxity of silver: implication for clinical wound care. *Burns* **30**(2): 140–7

Postmes T, Vandeputte J (1999) Recombinant growth factors or honey? *Burns* **25**: 676–8

Postmes TJ, Bosch MMC, Dutrieux R, van Baare J, Hoekstra MJ (1997) Speeding up the healing of burns with honey. An experimental study with histological assessment of wound biopsies. In: Mizrahi A, Lensky Y, eds. *Bee Products. Properties, Applications and Apitherapy*. Plenum Press, New York: 27–37

Rao GN, Berk BC (1992) Active oxygen species stimulate vascular smooth muscle cell growth and proto-oncogene expression. *Circ Res* **70**: 593–9

Richards L (2002) Healing infected recalcitrant ulcers with antibacterial honey. 4th Australian Wound Management Association Conference, Adelaide, Australia.

Robson V (2000) Personal communication. University Hospital Aintree, Liverpool, UK

Robson V, Dunford C, Molan PC, Cooper RA (2001) The use of honey in wound management. Innovations in Wound Care Conference, Cardiff, UK

Robson V, Ward RG, Molan PC (2000) The use of honey in split skin grafting. 10th Conference of the European Wound Management Association, Harrogate, UK

Ryan GB, Majno G (1977) *Inflammation*. Kalamazoo, Michigan, Upjohn

Schramm DD, Karim M, Schrader HR, Holt RR, Cardetti M, Keen CL (2003) Honey with high levels of antioxidants can provide protection to healthy human subjects. *J Agricultural Food Chemistry* **51**(6): 1732–35

Schreck R, Rieber P, Baeuerle PA (1991) Reactive oxygen intermediates as apparently widely used messengers in the activation of the NF-κB transcription factor and HIV-1. *EMBO J* **10**(8): 2247–58

Schultz GS, Sibbald RG, Falanga V, Ayello EA, Dowsett C, Harding K, Romanelli M, Stacey MC, Teot L, Vanscheidt W (2003) Wound bed preparation: a systematic approach to wound management. *Wound Rep Regen* **11** (suppl 1): s1–s28

Silver IA (1980) The physiology of wound healing. In: TK Hunt, *Wound Healing and Wound Infection: theory and surgical practice*. Appleton-Century-Crofts, New York: 11–28

Silvetti AN (1981) An effective method of treating long-enduring wounds and ulcers by topical applications of solutions of nutrients. *J Dermatol Surg Oncol* 7(6): 501–8

Sinclair RD, Ryan TJ (1994) Proteolytic enzymes in wound healing: the role of enzymatic debridement. *Aust J Dermatol* **35**: 35–41

Somerfield SD (1991) Honey and healing. *J R Soc Med* **84**(3): 179

Stewart J (2002) Therapeutic honey used to reduce pain and bleeding associated with dressing changes. 4th Australian Wound Management Association Conference, Adelaide, Australia

Subrahmanyam M (1991) Topical application of honey in treatment of burns. *Br J Surg* **78**(4): 497–8

Subrahmanyam M (1993) Honey-impregnated gauze versus polyurethane film (OpSite®) in the treatment of burns — a prospective randomised study. *Br J Plastic Surg* **46**(4): 322–3

Subrahmanyam M (1994) Honey-impregnated gauze versus amniotic membrane in the treatment of burns. *Burns* **20**(4): 331–3

Subrahmanyam M (1996) Honey dressing versus boiled potato peel in the treatment of burns: a prospective randomized study. *Burns* **22**(6): 491–3

Subrahmanyam M (1998) A prospective randomised clinical and histological study of superficial burn wound healing with honey and silver sulfadiazine. *Burns* **24**(2): 157–61

Subrahmanyam M, Sahapure AG, Nagane NS, Bhagwat VR, Ganu JV (2001) Effects of topical application of honey on burn wound healing. *Ann Burns Fire Disasters* **XIV**(3): 143–5

Suguna L, Chandrakasan G, Ramamoorthy U, Thomas Joseph K (1993) Influence of honey on biochemical and biophysical parameters of wounds in rats. *J Clin Biochemistry Nutrition* **14**: 91–9

Suguna L, Chandrakasan G, Thomas Joseph K (1992). Influence of honey on collagen metabolism during wound healing in rats. *J Clin Biochemistry Nutrition* **13**: 7–12

Taks JM (2000) Eusol managment of burns. *Trop Doct* **30**: 54

Tanaka H, Hanumadass M, Matsuda H, Shimazaki S, Walter RJ, Matsuda T (1995) Hemodynamic effects of delayed initiation of antioxidant therapy (beginning two hours after burn) in extensive third-degree burns. *J Burn Care Rehabil* **16**(6): 610–15

Tatnall FM, Leigh IM, Gibson JR (1991) Assay of antiseptic agents in cell culture: conditions affecting cytotoxicity. *J Hosp Infect* **17**(4): 287–96

Tur E, Bolton L, Constantine BE (1995) Topical hydrogen peroxide treatment of ischemic ulcers in the guinea pig: Blood recruitment in multiple skin sites. *J Am Acad Dermatol* **33**(2 Pt 1): 217–21

Vardi A, Barzilay Z, Linder N, Cohen HA, Paret G, Barzilai A (1998) Local application of honey for treatment of neonatal postoperative wound infection. *Acta Paediatr* **87**(4): 429–32

Viljanto J, Raekallio J (1976) Local hyperalimentation of open wounds. *Br J Surg* **63**: 427–30

Wadi M, Al-Amin H, Farouq A, Kashef H, Khaled SA (1987) Sudanese bee honey in the treatment of suppurating wounds. *Arab Medico* **3**: 16–18

Weheida SM, Nagubib HH, El-Banna HM, Marzouk S (1991) Comparing the effects of two dressing techniques on healing of low grade pressure ulcers. *J Med Research Institute*, Alexandria University **12**(2): 259–78

Weiss SJ, Peppin G, Ortiz X, Ragsdale C, Test ST (1985) Oxidative autoactivation of latent collagenase by human neutrophils. *Science* **227**: 747–9

White JW (1975). Composition of honey. In: Crane E, ed. *Honey: A comprehensive survey*. Heinemann, London: 157–206

Wood B, Rademaker M, Molan PC (1997) Manuka honey, a low cost leg ulcer dressing. *N Z Med J* **110**: 107

Zaiß (1934) Der Honig in äußerlicher Anwendung. *Münchener Medizinische Wochenschrift Nr* **49**: 1891–93

Zumla A, Lulat A (1989) Honey — a remedy rediscovered. *J R Soc Med* **82**(7): 384–5

CHAPTER 2

THE ANTIMICROBIAL ACTIVITY OF HONEY

Rose Cooper

It is now widely accepted that honey has antimicrobial activity and that this is dependent upon a variety of different modes of action (Molan, 1992a). These are known to include osmolarity, acidity, limited availability of water molecules, peroxide generation and antimicrobial chemicals. This chapter outlines the evidence for these different actions and illustrates how, even after dilution (as occurs upon interaction with wound exudate), the antimicrobial activity remains (Molan, 1992a, b).

Properties of honey that restrict microbial growth

All micro-organisms require supplies of nutrients that provide sources of carbon, nitrogen, minerals and water. Any restriction in the supply or availability of each key nutrient will tend to compromise microbial metabolism.

Honey contains approximately 80% sugar by weight, which is comprised of four main sugar molecules (fructose, glucose, maltose and sucrose), but with many others in lower quantities. The acids present in honey also help to restrict microbial growth. Complex mixtures of acids, particularly gluconic acid, contribute to low acidity and low pH (between 3.4 and 6.1) (White, 1979). These characteristics alone make all honeys unsuitable to support the growth of micro-organisms and explain why honeys destined for human consumption rarely spoil during storage in the home.

Honey is a super-saturated solution of sugars, with low water content, and the binding of water molecules to sugars makes them unavailable for micro-organisms. The availability of free water is expressed as water activity (A_w); pure water is A_w 1.00 and blood 0.99. Most honeys possess an A_w of approximately 0.6, and many microbial species require A_w between 0.94 and 0.99 to grow. The most osmotolerant bacteria (ie. those which can survive in high sugar concentration) are staphylococci; the minimum concentration of sucrose required to prevent growth of these bacteria is 29% (v/v) (Molan 1992a), at an A_w of 0.86 (Chirife _et al_, 1982).

Antimicrobial activity of honey

The first report of the antibacterial activity of honey has been attributed to a Dutch scientist, Van Ketel, in 1882 (Dustman, 1979). An indication that antimicrobial effects were not solely due to sugars came when Sackett (1919) showed that activity increased on dilution. Dold (1937) suggested the involvement of an antimicrobial substance termed 'inhibine', but the identity of the inhibine was not recognised until 1962, when Adcock demonstrated that catalase (an enzyme that degrades hydrogen peroxide) destroyed antibacterial activity. White _et al_ (1963) deduced that inhibine was hydrogen peroxide, which was generated by the action of glucose oxidase (an enzyme transferred from the hypopharyngeal glands of bees during nectar collection and honey processing in the hive). Levels of hydrogen peroxide are at undetectable levels in undiluted honeys because the enzyme is not active, but on dilution the uninhibited enzyme converts glucose into gluconic acid in the presence of oxygen. The rate of hydrogen peroxide generation on dilution in different honeys is not constant, and maximum levels of hydrogen peroxide were generated in honeys that were diluted by a factor of 2 to 3 (Bang _et al_, 2003).

The potency of the antibacterial activity of honeys shows marked differences (James _et al_, 1972; Molan _et al_, 1988; Al-Jabri _et al_, 2003). In a survey of 345 New Zealand unpasturised honeys from largely single floral sources, antibacterial activity was investigated using a bioassay based on an agar well diffusion technique (Allen _et al_, 1991). The extent of inhibition of a test bacterium (_Staphylococcus aureus_) was compared to that achieved by dilutions of phenol. Phenol (as carbolic acid) was the first antiseptic used in aseptic surgery and is an accepted reference chemical in evaluating disinfectants and antiseptics in laboratory tests.

In the New Zealand honeys, potency ranged from the equivalent of <2% (w/v) phenol to 58%, with significant differences between floral sources. When the test was performed with catalase added to the honey solutions, antibacterial activity disappeared from many honey samples, but was retained in only two types of honey tested, Manuka (*Leptospermum scoparium*) and viper's bugloss. Therefore, honeys with detectable activity were distinguished by their ability to generate hydrogen peroxide in the test (peroxide honeys), or their ability to retain potency in the presence of catalase (non-peroxide honeys). Some Australian non-peroxide honeys are known, for example, jellybush honey (*Leptospermum polygalifolium*). Since honeys do not significantly vary in their total sugar content (White *et al*, 1962), the antibacterial activity demonstrated in the bioassay used by Allen *et al* (1991) was attributed to either hydrogen peroxide or factors other than hydrogen peroxide. An example of a bioassay is presented in *Figure 2.1*.

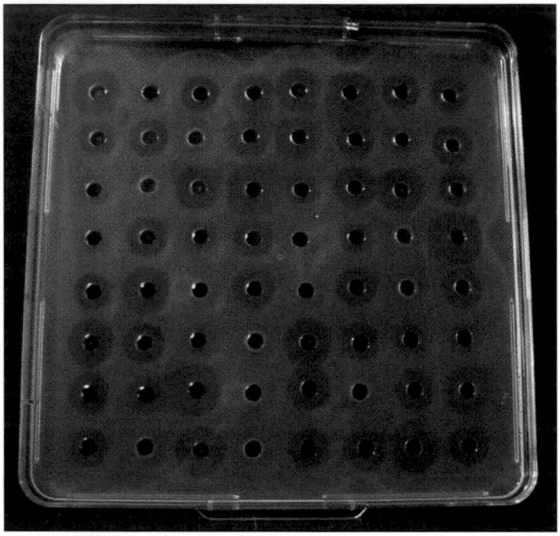

Figure 2.1: Bioassay to evaluate the antibacterial potency of honey. The clear zones show where bacteria that had been seeded into the agar have failed to grow. Wells contained diluted honey solutions or solutions of a range of concentrations of phenol

The nature of the non-peroxide antimicrobial activity of honeys

Despite numerous investigations into the nature of the non-peroxide components that confer antimicrobial activity to honey, definitive identifications and characterisations have not yet been published. The 'inhibine' mentioned earlier has been described as both a hydrogen peroxide activity and the effect of natural flavonoids and phenolic acids of plant origin (caffeic and ferulic acids) by Wahdan (1998).

The two readily identifiable sources of such components in honey are the bee and the floral source. A comparison of the antimicrobial activity of honey produced by a stingless bee and a honey bee in Costa Rica has suggested that plants, rather than bee species, influence potency (DeMera and Angert, 2004). However, Bogdanov (1997) suggested that both bee and plant influence activity. Phytochemicals, including the flavonoids, are secondary metabolites that confer colour, flavour and defence against infection to plants. Many possess antimicrobial potential and can be divided into several major groups (Cowan, 1999). The phenolic compounds and flavonoids have received the greatest attention, and these include some of the antioxidants known to be present in honeys. Separation of honey into four fractions showed Manuka to be exceptional in that most antibacterial activity was associated with the acidic fraction, whereas for other types of honey antibacterial activity was detected in all fractions (Bogdanov, 1997). Analysis of flavonoids in Swiss honeys indicated the presence of pinocembrin, which is an antimicrobial component characteristically found in another bee product, propolis or bee glue (Bogdanov, 1989). The phenolic components of ten Brazilian honeys have been extracted by HPLC and antibacterial activity evaluated. Compounds typical of Brazilian propolis were present in honeys, and geographical location was shown to influence chemical composition (Miorin _et al_, 2003). However, phenolic fractions of nineteen Manuka honeys neither varied with geographical location nor in their antibacterial potency (Weston _et al_, 2000). The antibacterial activity of high potency Manuka honey has been suggested to be associated with the carbohydrate fraction and not confined to the phenolic components (Weston _et al_, 1999).

The inhibition by honey of microbial species implicated in wound infections

More than a century after Van Ketel's observation, a comprehensive review of the inhibitory properties of honey was provided by Molan (1992a, b). By collating most of the previously published studies on the microbial species inhibited by honey, it could be seen that seventy-seven different species were inhibited by *in vitro* tests, but agreement about the susceptibilities of each species was absent. Comparisons between studies were impossible because varying techniques had been utilised, and descriptions of methods were incomplete or ambiguous; often neither the floral origin of the honey under investigation, nor detail of its processing was specified. Both heat and light can be shown to affect activity (Molan, 1992b), but these effects may not have been recognised in earlier studies.

Modern studies into the inhibition of wound pathogens by honey *in vitro* have confirmed its broad spectrum of activity, irrespective of whether honey was tested by being incorporated into broths (Willix *et al*, 1992; Karayil *et al*, 1998; Wahdan, 1998; Miorin *et al*, 2003), or agar plates (Nzeako and Hamdi, 2000; Subrahmanyam *et al*, 2001; Cooper *et al*, 2000; Cooper *et al*, 2002a, b; Blair, 2003). Using specified honeys of known potency, and comparing their antimicrobial activity to sugar solutions of similar osmolarity, some of these studies have confirmed that the activity of natural honeys is not solely attributable to their sugar content (Wahdan, 1998; Cooper *et al*, 2000; Cooper *et al*, 2002a, b; Blair, 2003). In many of these studies, Leptospermum honey, diluted by factors between 10 and 30, has inhibited test bacteria. It would not be expected that such low concentrations of honey would be used in wound care products, but the magnitude of the activity assures that dilution by wound exudates should not easily remove activity.

The mode of bacterial inhibition by honey has been seen to be bactericidal (killing), rather than bacteriostatic or growth-inhibiting (Wahdan, 1998; Cooper *et al* 2002a; Blair, 2003).

Antibiotic-resistant bacterial strains have been shown to be as susceptible to honeys as sensitive strains (Karayil *et al*, 1998; Cooper *et al*, 2000; Cooper *et al*, 2002a, b; Blair, 2003). Recent studies have, significantly, added methicillin-resistant *Staphylococcus aureus* (MRSA), vancomycin-resistant enterococci and *Burkholderia cepacia* (a pseudomonad-like bacterium associated with lung infection in cystic fibrosis with known resistance patterns) to the list of susceptible microbial species. Yeasts and fungi have also been reported to be susceptible to honey (Brady *et al*, 1996; Wahdan, 1998; Blair, personal communication).

At present, the mode of action of honey on bacterial cells has not yet been elucidated. An investigation into molecular effects using microarrays has indicated that the stress response is up-regulated in *Escherichia coli*, while some of the genes involved in protein synthesis are down-regulated (Blair, 2003). Morphological changes in bacteria exposed to Manuka honey (Cooper and Henriques, unpublished data), suggest that Gram positive and Gram negative bacteria do not respond identically. Further studies into cellular and molecular events are on-going.

The relevance of antimicrobial activity of honey to wounds

Polymicrobial communities are associated with wounds, but varying species may be found in different kinds of wounds (Bowler *et al*, 2001). The presence of micro-organisms in a wound may not necessarily be a cause for concern, since many do not give rise to infection. Routine application of antimicrobial agents to wounds can never be justified, because wounds do not have to be rendered sterile to heal successfully. There are complex interactions between the microbial inhabitants of wounds and human hosts that can result in differing outcomes, depending on microbial virulence and host immunocompetency. Infection, colonisation and contamination are three possible outcomes. Wound infection always interrupts the healing process and appropriate antimicrobial intervention is indicated. Guidelines for the selection of antibiotics in severe infections, and algorithms to manage hospital admissions are available (Eron *et al*, 2003). Nevertheless, rapid clearance of infection from honey-treated wounds that failed to respond to conventional therapies has been reported. The effectiveness of honey in limiting infection in burns patients was compared by Subrahmanyam (1998) to silver sulfadiazine. In this study, lower infection rates and faster healing was observed in those patients treated with honey.

Situations where topical agents are appropriate are not always immediately obvious; the reasons why wounds fail to heal are diverse and the involvement of micro-organisms is not yet entirely understood. The eradication from wounds of either β-haemolytic streptococci (Schraibman, 1990), or staphylococci and pseudomonads (Gilliland *et al*, 1988) before attempting skin grafting is accepted. The cases studies presented later in this book illustrate the clinical benefits of this activity.

In chronic wounds, the reduction of certain microbial species, such as anaerobic bacteria, has been advocated to limit undesirable odour (Bowler *et al*, 2001). Examples of clinical success where reduction of malodour was achieved have been reported (Dunford *et al*, 2000; Kingsley, 2001; and *Chapters 8* and 9 of this book).

MRSA-colonised wounds act as a potential reservoir of cross-infection, as well as having the potential to develop into an infection. Successful eradication of MRSA using honey has been achieved in reports of two patients to date (Dunford *et al*, 2000; Natarajan *et al*, 2001).

Conclusions

Already there is extensive laboratory evidence to demonstrate the antibacterial activity of honey, but to what degree this is relevant to the clinical situation can only be judged with its use. Certainly, reports of clinical studies tend to support the use of honey in reducing wound bioburden. Its broad spectrum of antimicrobial activity promises to make it an effective barrier to infection when applied to wounds, controlling ingress of environmental organisms, and, egress of wound pathogens. Many healthcare practitioners have been sceptical about the benefits of honey in managing wounds. It is encouraging to note the recent availability of CE marked products containing honey within the UK. More widespread use will ultimately provide the clinical evidence to prove or disprove previous claims.

References

Al-Jabri AA, Nzeako B, Al Mahrooqi *et al* (2003) In vitro antibacterial activity of Omani and African honey. *Br J Biomed Sci* **60**(1): 1–4

Allen KL, Molan PC, Reid GM (1991) A survey of the antibacterial activity of some New Zealand honeys. *J Pharm Pharmacol* **43**: 817–22

Adcock D (1962) The effect of catalase on the inhibine and peroxide values of various honeys. *J Apicult Res* **1**: 38–40

Bang LM, Bunting C, Molan PC (2003) The effect of dilution on the rate of hydrogen peroxide production in honey and its implications for wound healing. *J Altern Compl Med* **9**(2): 267–73

Blair SE (2003) *The therapeutic potential of honey*. PhD thesis. University of Sydney

Bogdanov S (1989) Determination of pinocembrin in honey using HPLC. *J Apicult Res* **28**(1): 55–7

Bogdanov S (1997) Nature and origin of the antibacterial substances in honey. *Lebensm Wiss u Technol* **30**: 748–53

Bowler PG, Duerden BJ, Armstrong DG (2001) Wound microbiology and associated approaches in wound management. *Clin Micro Rev* **14**(2): 244–69

Brady NF, Molan PC, Harfoot CG (1996) The sensitivity of dermatophytes to the antimicrobial activity of Manuka honey and other honey. *Pharm Sci* **2**: 1–3

Chirife J, Scarmato G, Herszage L (1982) Scientific basis for use of granulated sugar in treatment of infected wounds. *Lancet* **i**: 560–1

Cooper RA, Halas E, Molan PC (2002a) The efficacy of honey in inhibiting strains of *Pseudomonas aeruginosa* from infected burns. *J Burns Care Rehab* **23**: 366–70

Cooper RA, Molan PC, Harding KG (2002b) The sensitivity to honey of Gram-positive cocci of clinical significance isolated from wounds. *J Appl Micro* **93**: 857–63

Cooper RA, Wigley P, Burton NF (2000) Susceptibility of multiresistant strains of *Burkholderia cepacia* to honey. *Lett Appl Microbiol* **31**: 20–4

Cowan MM (1999) Plant products as antimicrobial agents. *Clin Micro Rev* **12**(4): 564–82

DeMera JH, Angert ER (2004) Comparison of the antimicrobial activity of honey produced by *Tetragonisca angustula* (Meliponinae) and *Apis mellifera* from different phytogeographic regions of Costa Rica. *Apidol* **35**: 411–17

Dunford CE, Cooper RA, Molan PC (2000) Using honey as a dressing for infected skin lesions. *Nurs Times* (NT Plus) **96**: 7–9

Dunford C, Cooper RA, Molan PC, White R (2000) The use of honey in wound management. *Nurs Standard* **29**: 63–7

Dustmann JH (1979) Antibacterial effect of honey. *Apiacta* **14**(1): 7–11

Eron LJ, Lipsky BA, Low DE., Nathwani D, Tice AD, Volturo GA (2003) Managing skin and soft tissue infections: expert panel recommendations on key decision points. *J Anti Chem* **52** (suppl 1): i3–17

Gilliland EL, Nathwani N, Dore CJ, Lewis JD (1988) Bacterial colonisation of leg ulcers and its effect on the success rate of skin grafting. *Ann R Coll Surg* **70**(2): 105–8

James OBO'L, Segree W, Ventura AK (1972) Some antibacterial properties of Jamaican honey. *W I Med J* **XXI** (7): 7–17

Karayil S, Deshpande SD, Koppikar GV (1998) Effect of honey on multidrug resistant organisms and its synergistic action with three common antibiotics. *J Postgrad Med* **44**: 93–7

Kingsley A (2001) The use of honey in the treatment of infected wounds: case studies. *Br J Nurs* (suppl) **10**(22): s13–s20

Miorin PL, Levy junior NC, Custodio AR, Bretz WA, Marcucci MC (2003) Antibacterial activity of honey and propolis from *Apis mellifera* and *Tetragonisca angustula* against *Staphylococcus aureus. J Appl Micro* **95**: 913–20

Molan PC (1992a) The antibacterial activity of honey. 1. The nature of the antibacterial activity. *Bee World* **73**: 5–28

Molan PC (1992b) The antibacterial activity of honey. 2. *Bee World* **73**: 59–76

Molan PC, Smith IM, Reid GM (1988) A comparison of some New Zealand honeys. *J Apic Res* **27**(4): 252–6

Natarajan S, Williamson D, Grey J, Harding KG, Cooper RA (2001) Healing of an MRSA-colonised, hydroxyurea-induced leg ulcer with honey. *J Dermat Treat* **12**: 33–6

Nzeako BC, Hamdi J (2000) Antimicrobial potential of honey on some microbial isolates. *Med Sci* **2**: 75–9

Sackett W.G. (1919) Honey as a carrier of intestinal diseases. *Bull Colo Agric Exp Stn No* 252: 18

Schraibman IG (1990) The clinical significance of β-haemolytic streptococci in chronic leg ulcers. *Ann Roy Coll Surg* **72**: 123–4

Subrahmanyam M (1998) A prospective randomised clinical and histological study of superficial burn wound healing with honey and silver sulphadiazine. *Burns* **24**: 157–61

Subrahmanyam M, Hemmady A, Pawar SG (2001) Antibacterial activity of honey on bacteria isolated from wounds. *Ann Burns Fire Dis* **XIV**(1): 22–4

Wahdan HA (1998) Causes of the antimicrobial activity of honey. *Infection* **26**(1): 26–31

Weston RJ, Brocklebank LK, Lu Y (2000) Identification and quantitative levels of antibacterial components of some New Zealand honeys. *Food Chem* **70**: 427–35

Weston RJ, Mitchell KR, Allen KL (1999) Antibacterial phenolic components of New Zealand manuka honey. *Food Chem* **64**: 295–301

White JW (1979) Composition of honey. In: Crane E, ed. *Honey: A comprehensive survey*. Heinemann, London: chap 5

White JW, Reithof ML, Subers MH, Kushnir I (1962) Comparison of American honeys. *Tech Bull US Dep Agric* **1261**: 124

White JW, Subers MH, Schepartz AI (1963) The identification of inhibine, the antibacterial factor in honey, as hydrogen peroxide and its origin in a honey glucose-oxidase system. *Biochem Biophys Acta* **73**: 57–70

Willix DJ, Molan PC, Harfoot CG (1992) A comparison of the sensitivity of wound-infecting species of bacteria to the antibacterial activity of Manuka honey and other honey. *J Appl Bact* **73**: 388–94

Chapter 3

Implications of honey dressings within primary care

Jackie Stephen-Haynes

Introduction

The challenge of wound care within the primary care setting relates to two key areas: healing or managing symptoms. While the objective would ideally be healing, chronic wound management hinges on managing symptoms. Honey has been used historically for its therapeutic properties, including, the promotion of rapid wound healing, reducing oedema, debriding necrotic tissue, reducing inflammation, stimulating tissue regeneration as a topical treatment for infected wounds (Molan, 2002; Vander Weyden, 2003), and can be effective on antibiotic resistant strains of bacteria (Molan, 1992; Cooper and Molan, 1999; Cooper *et al*, 1999; Dunford *et al*, 2000). Therefore, the effectiveness of honey should be judged on the purpose for the intervention, whilst acknowledging the additional components.

Pure honey is a semi-translucent concentrated mixture of glucose, fructose, proteins, fatty acids, minerals, vitamins and water produced by worker bees from the nectar of flowers. Honey varies due to the pollen content and floral source from which it is obtained. Nectar is a weak natural sugar solution that the bees convert through enzymatic action into honey, which is stored in cells within the hive and covered with a thick waxy substance (beeswax) as a food store.

Until now, honey has not been developed and specified as a wound management product, and has not been regulated by pharmaceutical or Medical Device standards. The first honey dressing available on FP10 (UK prescription) was Activon™ tulle (Advancis Medical), which is a low adherent sterile dressing, impregnated with 20–25g of Manuka honey per 10 cm x 10 cm and 5–6g per 5 cm x 5 cm dressing. New dressings combining honey with a functional 'carrier' are becoming available; for example, honey with alginate or hydrogel sheet. This offers an ancillary action such as extra exudate handling capacity in the case of alginate-honey combination.

To safeguard the patient and act in accordance with the Nursing and Midwifery Council (NMC) (2002), it is important that only products that are a pharmaceutical device or available as CE Medical Devices are used on patients. This is particularly important in relation to honey dressings, as they are easily available from non-medical sources in a non-sterile form. It is essential that honey used for medicinal purposes is pure and free from synthetic pesticides. Some honey contains phytochemicals associated with anti-bacterial activity (Molan 2001). Honey from Manuka has a high level of these (Allen *et al*, 1991) and, as such, is among the highest potency honey available in the world. Manuka is the local Maori name for the New Zealand tea tree *Leptospermum scoparium*. Australian honey is reported to have a less effective antimicrobial effect (Molan, 2001), but further research would be needed to confirm or refute this.

Honey may, therefore, be a useful addition to the current range of products as it has several attributes (Molan, 1999):

* ⌘ Antimicrobial
* ⌘ Deodorisation
* ⌘ Debriding
* ⌘ Anti-inflammatory
* ⌘ Stimulation of new tissue growth

Antimicrobial activity

Chronic wounds, such as leg ulcers and pressure ulcers, are commonly infected or heavily colonised with bacteria (Scanlon and Stubbs, 2002; Booth, 2003). Much of the research about honey is related to its anti-bacterial properties (Molan, 1992; Cooper and Molan, 1999; Cooper *et al*, 1999; Dunford *et al*, 2000).

While clinical criteria for identifying wound infection has been identified by Cutting and Harding (1994), this is considered too generic (Cutting and White, 2004), and healthcare professionals are encouraged to consider the major categories of wounds separately to avoid overlooking the possibility of infection. Indeed, determining infected and non-infected wounds has become more complicated as other criteria for recognising infection are increasingly recognised. Certainly, the 'granulating' or 'red' wound may be healing in a normal way, or may appear as red when infected with haemolytic streptococci (Gray _et al_ 2003). With the recognition of terms such as 'critically colonised', a wound swab is no longer conclusive that a wound is free from infection. Although the wound swab may be negative, there is delayed healing with a host reaction, which commonly responds to an antimicrobial dressing such as iodine, silver or honey. These differentiations are not easily defined by microbiological characterisation or quantification, and practitioners find it increasingly difficult to differentiate in clinical practice. The Wound Infection Continuum, as part of applied wound management, is useful (Kingsley, 2001a; White, 2003b).

Colonisation   Critical colonisation   Local infection   Systemic infection

The Wound Infection Continuum

The following criteria for wound infection should also be utilised as a guide (Cutting and Harding, 1994):

- abscess
- cellulitis
- discharge
- delayed healing
- discolouration
- friable, bleeding granulation tissue
- unexpected pain or tenderness
- pocketing, bridging at base of wound
- abnormal smell
- wound breakdown.

Systemic antibiotics are indicated for those with clinical infections, whilst the use of topical antibiotics is generally avoided because of the increase in bacterial resistance (Cooper and Lawrence, 1996). The use of antiseptics is controversial (Scanlon and Stubbs, 2002), as they are non-selective and can be toxic to the host tissue (Booth, 2003). More recently in the UK, the emphasis has been on the use of antimicrobial dressings, which currently account for several million in the UK.

The most commonly used antimicrobial dressings are silver (White, 2003a; Lansdown, 2003) and iodine, which is a topical germicidal agent, effective against bacteria, fungi and protozoa (Hansson, 2001). Despite the availability of these in an increasingly wide range of applications (alginates, foams, lipido-colloids), patients frequently ask about using honey and a surprising number present with Internet searches on honey. The emergence of 'antibiotic resistance', and the growing interest in 'natural' or 'complementary' therapies, has led to an interest in honey dressings. The anti-bacterial effect of honey is related to a number of its properties, including; pH, osmolarity, phytochemicals and the production of hydrogen peroxide. The pH of honey is characteristically between 3.2 and 4.5 and is low enough to inhibit pathogens such as *E.coli*, *Pseudomonas spp*, *Salmonella spp* and *Streptococcus pyogenes* (Molan, 2001).

The anti-bacterial effects of Manuka honey are also assisted by the presence of hydrogen peroxide, an oxidising agent released by the action of the enzyme peroxidase. Hydrogen peroxide is considered unsafe at a high level (Booth, 2003) with a bleaching action that may cause pain (Lawrence, 1997). In honey dressings, hydrogen peroxide is at a very low level (1000 times less than in 3% hydrogen peroxide), is still an effective antibacterial agent (Ambrose *et al*, 1991) and compatible with cellular preservation (Booth, 2003). Healing depends much upon creating equilibrium between host defence mechanisms and the multitude of pathological organisms that occur in the wound environment (Lansdown, 2003).

Topically, hydrogen peroxide removes contaminants, cleanses and de-odorises wounds and stimulates macrophage vascular endothelial growth factor, which is released in the initial inflammatory stages of wound healing (Cho *et al*, 2001). Hydrogen peroxide is naturally produced by the body in the cells as a result of glucose metabolism, and is considered to be non-toxic to the host tissue (Booth, 2003). The application of hydrogen peroxide with a similar level to the natural level may trigger responses in the chronic wound, and may restart the healing process. When honey is diluted and applied to the wound it produces hydrogen peroxide at a steady rate, providing a sustained, effective delivery (Booth, 2003). *In vitro* studies support the antimicrobial effect of honey against a wide range of pathogens including beta-haemolytic streptococci, MRSA and *Pseudomonas spp* (Allen *et al*, 1991; Cooper and Molan, 1999). The *in vivo* studies are less conclusive, but honey has been used to treat burns (Efem, 1988), meningococcal lesions (Dunford *et al*, 2000), venous leg ulcers, pressure ulcers, diabetic foot ulcers, donor sites, abscesses and boils (Betts and Molan, 2001). Subrahmanyan (1998) compared honey to silver sulfadiazine and found less inflammation, lower infection rates, and faster healing in burns patients treated with honey.

The anti-bacterial action may also be responsible for honey's anti-inflammatory effect as well as stimulating new tissue growth (Molan 1999). Conversely, (Kingsley, 2001b) reports two case studies where honey failed to eliminate infection, and Alcaraz and Kelly (2002) report that honey failed to eliminate bacteria from a chronic wound. However, Alcaraz and Kelly (2002) did find an improvement in managing exudate and de-odourisation.

In 1892, Van Ketel (Molan, 2001) noted the high osmolarity of honey, and Cooper (1999) reported that it continued to prevent the growth of _Staphylococcus aureus_ when diluted seven to fourteen times. However, this high osmolarity may be reduced in the presence of exudate until it can no longer inhibit infection (Molan, 2001).

This poses the question of whether the evidence indicates that honey dressings should be used in an infected wound, one that is critically colonised, or, for patients who are at risk of developing an infection. Further research is needed and this should be a primary area for focus. The potential for honey may be lost by inadequate research reporting where any honey is evaluated rather than specific honey. The variance in the antimicrobial effect is important and within clinical practice there is a need to ensure that appropriate honey is applied. The case of 'honey in the jar' being effective is largely anecdotal and not reported in the literature

Deodorising and debriding

Van der Weyden (2003) reports using honey alginate on two patients with pressure ulcers, which led to rapid and complete healing in both wounds and noted a de-odorising and anti-inflammatory effect. Honey is now used as standard treatment in chronic wounds within this particular nursing home. Lisle (2002) reports the use of sugar paste being effective in a single care study. Similarly, Stephen-Haynes (2004) reports case studies where debridement of wounds with three patients and management of odour in five patients occurred. There is clearly a need for the control of malodorous wounds (Scanlon and Stubbs, 2002; Booth, 2003). Hampton (2004) identifies the importance of this with patients with fungating wounds, and recognises the role that community staff will have in providing the care.

Anti-inflammatory and stimulation of new tissue growth

Topham (2002) highlights the effect that honey has on the extra-cellular matrix, and Dunford *et al* (2000) reports significant epithelialisation when honey was used. Marshall (2002) reports the use of honey in podiatry and Templeton (2002) reports the reduction of inflammation and the stimulation of angiogenesis and the formation of granulation tissue. However, the small scales of their research are acknowledged and the need for further exploratory research highlighted.

Dressing selection in clinical practice — choosing honey

The current trend within tissue viability is to consider the concept of wound bed preparation (Falanga, 2000), as well as other traditional factors (Stephen Haynes and Gibson, 2003). Implementing this in clinical practice has been assisted by the development of the acronym TIME: tissue, infection, moisture, and edge (Schultz *et al*, 2003). This has implications for wound management (Dowsett and Ayello, 2004)

Factors to consider in relation to dressing selection (Stephen Haynes and Gibson, 2003) include:

- wound classification
- stage of healing
- aetiology
- tissues involved
- level of exudate
- level of pain
- the peri-wound area
- the patient's general health and environment
- cost-effectiveness of the dressing.

The criteria of an ideal dressing (Turner, 1985), include:

- keeping wound moist
- managing exudate
- allowing gaseous exchange
- thermal insulation of the wound
- protecting from contamination
- protecting from micro-organisms
- protecting the wound from trauma.

Wound bed preparation and T.I.M.E. (Schultz *et al* 2003)

❖ T	Tissue	Tissue non-viable or deficient
❖ I	Infection	Infection or inflammation
❖ M	Moisture	Moisture imbalance
❖ E	Edge	Edge of wound, non-advancing or undermined

It may be useful to consider the mode of honey application in relation to these factors. Assessing the patient and the wound will highlight holistic factors as, in most clinical situations, honey may not be the only active intervention that needs to be employed to effect a result, for example, antibiotics, pressure relief, bed rest, limb elevation and compression bandaging.

The Infection Continuum (White, 2003b) is useful in raising awareness of 'critical colonisation', which may delay healing and, therefore, may be an indicator for an antimicrobial dressing such as honey. The Wound Healing Continuum (Gray *et al*, 2003) offers a useful framework for assessment and classification, and utilising the concept of TIME (Schultz *et al*, 2003) assists with identifying the aim of wound management.

By clearly assessing the wound, the objective can be determined and the mode of application of honey can be considered.

Infection Continuum

Colonisation   Critical colonisation   Local infection   Systemic infection

Wound Healing Continuum

Necrotic, necrotic/sloughy, sloughy, sloughy/granulating, granulating/epithelialisation and epithelialisation

TIME

Tissue   Inflammation-Infection   Moisture   Edge

Debride and restore wound base, remove infection, restore epithelial migration, advancing edge

Application of mode of honey

Ointment/gel honey   Honey + alginate   Honey tulle   Honey + foam/film

Dressing evaluation

A preliminary report of this evaluation has previously been reported in the *British Journal of Nursing* (Stephen-Haynes, 2004).

Some reports on the effectiveness of honey relate to 'generic honey' of an unspecified source. Advancis Medical produce an impregnated non-adherent dressing, which contains Manuka honey. Although honey dressings have been available, they have not been under pharmaceuticals devices or available as CE Medical Devices. The contraindications to the use of honey dressings are allergy to honey and allergy to bee venom. The dressing may be used in patients with diabetes, but they should be monitored closely for absorbency of glucose.

Study method

An evaluation has been undertaken in the Worcestershire primary care trusts. This evaluation contains analysis of Activon™ Tulle (Advancis Medical), which is sterile, non-adherent and impregnated with 20–25g of Manuka honey. The dressing is applied directly to the wound and then secured with bandaging or film, possibly in conjunction with absorbent padding. The lack of evidence of specific wound types that benefit from honey dressings led to all classification of wounds being included in the Wound Healing Continuum (Gray *et al*, 2003), any classification within the Infection Continuum (White, 2003b), and any objective in TIME (Schultz *et al*, 2003). The factors considered were:

- wound position and size
- ease of application and removal
- whether the dressing stayed in place
- management of exudate
- patient comfort
- wound bed condition.

The assessment of each patient included:

- patient demographic information: age, gender, height-weight, body mass index (BMI)
- diabetes

- anaemia
- nutritional status (Russell, 2002)
- pressure ulcer risk assessment (Waterlow, 1985, 2005).

Each wound was assessed (Stephen-Haynes and Gibson, 2003), the dimensions recorded, and photographs were taken with consent from the patient.

Results

Analysis is made of twenty patient episodes with statistical data presented in a chart (*Figure 3.1*).

Of the twenty patients: eleven presented with leg ulceration, two mixed aetiology, one arterial and eight venous (representing a typical percentage of patients commonly seen in practice with each leg ulcer aetiology), one foot ulcer, two burns, two pressure ulcers, one with an injury to the knee, two traumatic skin tears and one drainage of haematoma.

Ease of application

Sixty-five per cent of the evaluations considered the dressing easy to apply, and 30% found it to be average or on a par with other dressings. Five per cent found the application difficult. Such differentiation may relate to the size of the dressing. The dressing is now available as a 10 cm x 10 cm and a 5 cm x 5 cm, which should help application. The 5 cm x 5 cm size is a particularly useful addition for patients with toe/toenail wounds and should be an area of further research.

Ease of removal

Seventy-five per cent evaluated the dressing as being easily removed and 25% found it to be average. All the comments were positive in relation to the ease of removal, and it was considered to be an 'atraumatic' dressing.

Patient	Age	Wound type	Wound classification	Allergies
1	72	Leg ulcer	Sloughy	None
2	83	Mixed aetiology leg ulcer	Granulating/sloughy	None
3	75	Chronic leg ulcer	Granulating	Has reacted to some products
4	89	Ischaemic ulcer	Granulating	None
5	90	Venous leg ulcer	Slough	None
6	76	Venous ulcer	Slough/granulating	Hydrocolloids
7	88	Mixed aetiology leg ulcer	Infected	None
8	75	Venous leg ulcer	Sloughy	None
9	78	Foot ulcer		Granuflex and iodine
10	88	Burn	Granulating	None
11	70	Traumatic skin tear	Granulating	None
12	89	Pressure ulcer grade 2	Slough	None
13	88	Burn	Slough	None
14	68	Injury to left knee	Granulating	Iodine
15	68	Drainage of haematoma	Sloughy	None
16	75	Venous leg ulcer	Sloughy	None
17	69	Laceration to lower leg	Granulating/sloughy	None
18	84	Venous leg ulcer	Sloughy	None
19	58	Traumatic wound	Granulating/sloughy	None
20	72	Pressure ulcer	Granulating/sloughy	None

Figure 3.1: Chart of patient characteristics

Dressing staying in place

Eighty-five per cent of evaluations found the dressing stayed in place as long as recommended. Fifteen per cent found the dressing did not last as long as recommended. This may be related to the level of exudates, and the addition of an alginate component would assist with this. The dressing surface in contact with wound bed is essentially in a fluid state, which means the dressing can be easily lifted off the wound without sticking, and any excess honey easily rinsed away.

Improvement in wound bed

Eighty per cent found an improvement in the wound bed, whilst 20% did not. However, the practitioner needs to consider the objective of using the honey dressing.

Patient comfort

Sixty-five per cent found it to be comfortable, 15% fairly comfortable and 20% found it uncomfortable. It was noted that pain subsided after the first dressing change. The patient may experience a drawing or stinging sensation due to the high osmolarity of the honey. This reduces the water activity of micro-organisms to a level where they are either inert or destroyed.

Wound dressings can be traumatic to the wound bed and the peri-wound area. Controlling pain at dressing change (Hollinworth, 2000) and being an 'atraumatic' dressing (Thomas, 2003) are important criteria. The practitioner should be mindful of pain when considering the application of honey dressings and should advise the patient on an appropriate course of action.

Three individual case studies are included which highlight the results seen within clinical practice.

Case study 1

Mrs H is an eighty-eight-year-old lady who has had lower leg ulceration of mixed aetiology for many years, and whose care is shared between a vascular consultant and a district nursing team. Mrs H is registered blind, has a history of osteo-arthritis and has been wheelchair-bound for approximately thirty years. There have been many episodes of non-concordance regarding her treatment/medication, which have challenged both medical and nursing staff.

Mrs H had previously been treated with high compression bandaging (Tensopress™, Smith and Nephew Limited) and visited the vascular consultant every three months. A holistic assessment of Mrs H was carried out by the district nurse upon admission to the caseload, and she was found to be anaemic and suffering from hypothyroidism, both of which were corrected by her GP.

A wound assessment was completed and Doppler ultrasound was attempted but was unsuccessful, therefore a re-assessment by the vascular team was requested, as, at this time, the ulcers on both lower legs showed signs of deterioration. Following an MRI scan both legs were found to have arterial components that required surgical intervention. An angioplasty was partially successful to the left

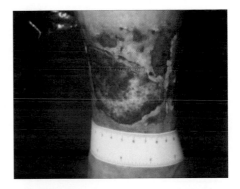

Figure 3.2a: Back of the left lower leg, 17/3/03

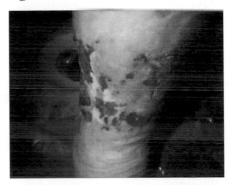

Figure 3.2b: Front of the left lower leg, 17/3/03

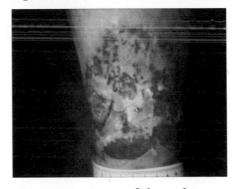

Figure 3.2c: Front of the right lower leg, 17/3/03

leg but unsuccessful to the right (further appropriate surgery is presently being discussed). Over many years various dressings have been used with limited success and, more recently, peri-wound maceration due, in part, to non-concordance of diuretic therapy and high limb elevation had become a real problem as there was marked lower leg oedema.

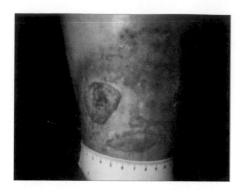

Figure 3.2d: Anterio-lateral side of right lower leg, 24/3/03

In considering the continuums, being a leg ulcer it is likely to be at least colonised (Scanlon and Stubbs, 2002), and with the appearance of slough/granulation tissue, it may be critically colonised, explaining the non-healing. The aim on the TIME continuum would be to remove infection. The size of the wound and the level of exudate was such that the addition of an alginate would be beneficial. Honey could be applied with a honey and alginate dressing.

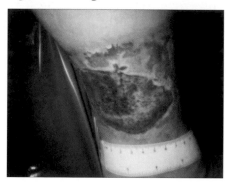

Figure 3.2e: Back of the left lower leg, 24/3/03

Photographs of both legs were taken prior to first application and at weekly intervals for the first month. Activon™ Tulle (Advancis Medical) was applied to the ulcers on both legs, and extended to cover all of the surrounding badly macerated skin. Daily dressing changes took place initially but, as removal of slough and surrounding skin and the condition of both the ulcer beds improved, these were reduced to alternate days and eventually twice a week.

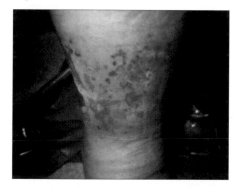

Figure 3.2f: Front of the left lower leg, 24/3/03

The dressing was easy to apply and remove but the initial application caused some discomfort, and stinging. This caused an unsettled first night despite regular analgesia; however, Mrs H was determined to continue with the treatment and subsequent applications of the dressing caused much lower levels of discomfort that settled half-an-hour after application.

The rapid improvement in the peri-wound skin was quite dramatic over the first four weeks, with the initial affected areas of over 10 cm square healing completely, and improvement in the wound beds of each ulcer. Patient concordance of both high elevation and prescribed

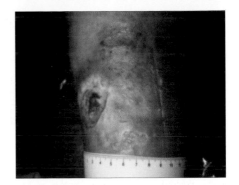

Figure 3.2g: Front of the right lower leg, 31/3/03

medication improved over the trial period (this could have contributed, in part, to the dramatic improvement in such a short period of time).

Mrs H's ulcers and badly macerated surrounding skin responded well to treatment during the first four weeks. All broken skin adjacent to both ulcers healed and the ulcer beds looked much healthier than they had done pre-trial evaluation. No wound swabs were taken during this case study, so the antimicrobial effect cannot be corroborated.

Case study 2

Mrs A is aged eighty-eight years and mobile. She sustained a burn on her left upper arm following a fall onto an electric fire. The area measured 20 cm x 15 cm and had been allowed to dry out.

In considering the continuums, the wound appeared necrotic, sloughy (Gray *et al*, 2003), and infected with MRSA (White, 2003b). The treatment objectives were to manage infection and to debride the wound (Schulz *et al*, 2003).

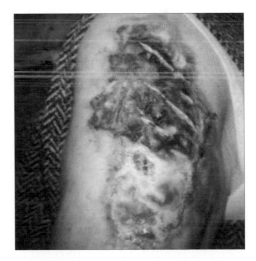

Figure 3.1: Mrs A as at 28 February, 2003

Initial treatment with hydrogel aimed to soften and promote autolysis to remove the eschar. Wound swab showed MRSA infection, which was treated systemically with amoxacillin and flucloxacillin. Mrs A found treatment distressing and, following one and a half weeks of hydrogel treatment, little progress had been made. The eschar remained dry, causing the wound to be tight and painful. Mrs A agreed to evaluate Activon™ Tulle honey with the aim of promoting autolysis and preventing the re-occurrence of infection. Softening of the eschar was seen within a week and the wound was less painful. Within three weeks the wound was visibly debriding. Within ten weeks, total debridement had taken place, and there were visible signs of large areas of epithelialisation. Mrs A found this dressing comfortable to wear and never experienced any pain following application.

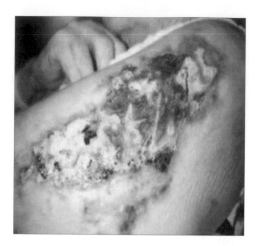

Figure 3.2: Mrs A as at 7 March, 2003

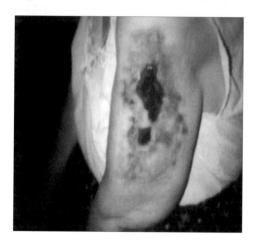

Figure 3.3: Mrs A as at 9 May, 2003

Case study 3

Mrs J is eighty-nine years old. She was admitted for rehabilitation following bilateral cellulitus, which had led to reduced mobility. She is obese and presented with a broken area on her left calf, measuring 6 cm x 2 cm. In considering the continuums, the wound (Gray *et al,* 2003) appeared sloughy with minimal exudate with macerated peri–wound area. The wound was not infected and would be classified as colonised (White, 2003b). The aim of the treatment on the TIME continuum

(Schultz *et al,* 2003) would be to prevent infection, and promote granulation. As she was allergic to iodine and topical antimicrobial therapy was indicated, treatment with honey was commenced and the wound healed in approximately four weeks. No pain was reported; the dressing was comfortable and was easily removed.

Conclusion

Clinical governance and evidence-based practice are now an important element of delivering care in the NHS (DoH, 1997). To safeguard the patient and act in accordance with the NMC (2002), it is important that only those products that are a pharmaceuticals device or available as CE Medical Devices are used on patients. This is particularly important in relation to honey dressings, as they are easily available from non-medical sources in a non-sterile form. The existing evidence on honey is largely based on *in vivo* studies, with no confirmation from a well-designed clinical trial.

Perhaps the only relevant studies on the likely usefulness are those undertaken with standardised honey (Molan, 2001). Nevertheless, the mounting evidence suggests that honey has an increasingly important role in wound care, which will be welcomed by the patient who increasingly seeks a 'natural' approach to wound care. The increasing concerns relating to antibiotic resistance, as well as the safety or toxicity of topical antiseptics, provides the impetus to search for a safe agent that can assist in the management of infected and critically colonised wounds, and in the prevention of infection. While an evaluation in clinical practice has limited generalisability, there is a value in any evaluation that is *in vivo* rather than *in vitro*.

The use of antiseptics always needs careful consideration and justification (*Chapter 2*). Honey provides sustained release of hydrogen peroxide at a level which is non-toxic (*Chapter 2*). It also has the ability to manage exudate, debride wounds and be comfortable on the wound (*Chapter 9*). At the time of writing, there are a number of honey-based wound treatments with the CE mark which are available on prescription.

Careful monitoring for any allergic responses or the dressing being an irritant are key concerns. The dressing should not be used by those allergic to honey or bee venom. There may be a risk of hyperglycaemia and the patient will need to be monitored closely.

Based on the experience gathered in these cases, it is clear that honey meets many of the criteria of the ideal dressing (Turner, 1985).

The future

Much needed, further research with honey in the clinical arena is being undertaken, particularly in relation to its role in infection/colonisation and its use as a podiatry dressing. There is a need for evidence from clinical practice to guide future practice and the development of an educational strategy for its use. It is essential that patients with diabetes are included in its usage, and are monitored closely.

The financial cost of infected wounds in the UK may also be a considerable force in the future development of honey dressings. For example, will we soon be witnessing a plethora of dressings and modes of application of honey as we have witnessed with silver? Will we be witnessing a foam dressing impregnated with honey, or a hydrocolloid and honey, or aqueous cream and honey?

While a randomised controlled trial (RCT) or controlled study is needed to guide future practice, those with responsibility for formularies for dressing selection should consider this product as an additional effective wound management product, rather than as an 'alternative treatment', as it has a significant role in wound bed preparation and total care of the patient.

References

Alcaraz A, Kelly J (2002) Treatment of an infected venous leg ulcer with honey dressings. *Br J Nurs* **11**(13): 859–66

Allen K, Molan P, Reid G (1991) A survey of the antibacterial activity of some New Zealand honeys. *J Pharmacol* **43**(12): 817–82

Ambrose U, Middleton K, Seal D (1991) In vitro studies of water activity and bacterial growth inhibition of sucrose-polyethylene glycol 400-hydrogen peroxide and xylose-polyethylene glycol 400-hydrogen peroxide pastes used to treat wounds. *Antimicrobial agents chemotherapy* **35**(9): 799–1803

Booth S (2003) Are honey and sugar paste alternatives to topical antiseptics? *J Wound Care* **13**(1): 31–3

Betts J, Molan P (2001) A pilot trial of honey as a wound dressing has shown the importance of the way honey is applied to the wounds. 11th conference of the European Wound Management Association. Dublin, Ireland

Cho M, Hunt T, Hussain M (2001) Hydrogen peroxide stimulates vascular endothelial growth factor release. *Am J Physiol* **280**: 5

Cooper R, Lawrence J (1996) Microorganisms and wounds. *J Wound Care* **5**(5): 233–6

Cooper R, Molan P (1999) The use of honey as an antiseptic in managing *pseudomonas* infection. *J Wound Care* **8**(4): 161–4

Cooper R, Molan PC, Hardking KG (1999) Antibacterial activity of honey against strains of *Staphylococcus aureus* from infected wounds. *J R Soc Med* **92**(6): 283–5

Cutting K, White R (2004) Defined and refined: criteria for identifying wound infection re-visited. *Br J Community Nurs* **9**(3) (suppl): s6–s15

Cutting K, Harding K (1994) Criteria for identifying wound infection. *J Wound Care* **3**(4): 198–201

Department of Health (1997) *The new NHS modern, dependable.* DoH, London

Dowsett C, Aayello E (2004) TIME principles of chronic wound bed preparation and treatment. *Br J Nurs* (Tissue Viability supplement) **13**(15): s16–s21

Dunford C, Cooper R, Molan P, White R (2000) The use of honey in wound management. *Nurs Standard* **15**(11): 63–8

Efem S (1988) Clinical observations of the wound healing properties of honey. *Br J Surg* **75**(7): 679–81

Falanga V (2000) Classification for wound bed preparation and stimulation of chronic wounds. *Wound Repair Regen* **8**(5): 347–52

Gray D, White R, Cooper P (2003) The wound healing continuum. In White RJ, ed. *The Silver Book.* Quay Books, MA Healthcare Limited, London: 1–12

Hampton S (2004) Managing symptoms of fungating wounds. *J Community Nurs* **18**(10): 22–6

Hansson C (2001) Iodine therapy. In: Cherry G, Harding K, Ryan T, eds. *Wound Bed Preparation. International congress and symposium.* Royal Society of Medicine Press Ltd, London: chap 7, pp 49–52

Hollinworth H (2000) Pain and wound care. *Wound Care Society Educational Leaflet* **7**(2) May

Kingsley A (2001a) A proactive approach to wound infection. *Nurs Standard* **15**(30): 50–8

Kingsley A (2001b) The use of honey in the treatment of infected wounds: case studies. *Br J Nurs* **22**(10): 12–20

Lansdown A (2003) Silver in wound care and management. *Wound Care Society Educational Booklet* **11**(3)

Lawrence J (1997) Wound irrigation. *Wound Care* **6**(1): 23–6

Lisle J (2002) Use of sugar in the treatment of infected leg ulcers. *Br J Community Nurs* **7**(6) (suppl): 40–6

Marshall C (2002) The use of honey in wound care: a review article. *Br J Podiatry* **5**(2): 47–9

Molan P (1992) The anti bacterial activity of honey: 1. The nature of the antibacterial activity. *Bee World* **73**(1): 5–28

Molan P (1999) The role of honey in the management of wounds. *J Wound Care* **8**(8): 415–18

Molan P (2001) Honey as a topical antibacterial agent for treatment of infected wounds. Available online at: www.worldwidewounds.com

Molan P (2002) Re-introducing honey in the management of wounds and ulcers: theory and practice. *Ostomy Wound Management* **48**(11): 28–40

Nursing and Midwifery Council (2002) *Nursing and Midwifery Code of Professional Conduct*. NMC, London.

Russell L (2002) The importance of wound documentation and classification. In: White R, ed. *Trends in Wound Care*, volume one. Quay Books, MA Healthcare Limited, London

Scanlon E, Stubbs N (2002) To use or not to use? The debate on the use of antiseptics in wound care. *Br J Community Nurs* **7**(9) (suppl): s8–s20

Schultz G, Sibbald G, Falanga V *et al* (2003) Wound bed preparation: a systematic approach to wound management. *Wound Rep Regen* **11**(2): 1–28

Stephen-Haynes J, Gibson E (2003) Anatomy, physiology wound healing and wound assessment. *Wound Care Society Educational Booklet* **1**(2)

Stephen-Haynes (2004) Evaluation of honey-impregnated tulle dressing in primary care. *Br J Community Nurs* **9**(6) (suppl): s21–s27

Subrahmanyam M (1998) A prospective, randomised clinical and histological study of superficial burn wound healing with honey and silver sulphadiazine. *Burns* **24**(2): 157–61

Templeton S (2002) A review of the use of honey in wounds. *ACCNS J Community Nurses* **7**(1): 13–14

Thomas S (2003) Atraumatic dressings. World wide wounds. Available online at: www.worldwidewounds

Topham J (2002) Why do some cavity wounds treated with honey or sugar paste heal without scarring? *J Wound Care* **11**(2): 53–5

Turner T (1985) Which dressing and why. In: Westaby S, ed. *Wound Care*. Heinemann, London

van der Weyden E (2003) The use of honey for the treatment of two patients with pressure ulcers. *Br J Community Nurs* **8**(12) (suppl): s14–s20

Waterlow J (1985) Pressure sores: a risk assessment card. *Nurs Times* **81**(48): 49–95

Waterlow J (2005) *Pressure Ulcer Prevention Manual*. Revised. Available online from: www.judy-waterlow.co.uk

White R (2003a) An historical overview of the use of silver in wound management. In: White R, ed. *The Silver Book*. Quay Books, MA Healthcare Limited, London

White R (2003b) The wound infection continuum. In: White R, ed. *Trends in Wound Care*, volume 2. Quay Books, MA Healthcare Limited, London

CHAPTER 4

PRACTICAL USE OF MODERN HONEY DRESSINGS IN CHRONIC WOUNDS

Andrew Kingsley

Choosing to use a honey dressing

As with any other dressing product, the choice of honey as a wound dressing product must be linked to the properties ascribed to it. Nor is it different with respect to gaining informed consent from the patient. The practitioner using it needs to be knowledgeable about the benefits and the problems of application to negotiate a care plan with the patient. This aspect of negotiation may come into sharp focus, as products that could be considered alternative or complementary by some, can lead to vociferous demands for use by the patient. From the author's experience to date, honey appears to be associated with positive attitudes and interest by patients when it has been introduced into discussion as a treatment possibility. For those patients who request honey, it can be necessary to temper a degree of over-optimism about outcomes with realism gained from clinical practice: expectations of 'miracle cures' have a tendency to disappoint in the field of chronic wound healing. In this situation, patients have usually purchased a non-medical grade honey from a health-food shop, so it may be necessary to discuss sensitively the pros and cons of this and, in some cases, source a suitable alternative honey product for use.

Molan (1999) describes the following key therapeutic attributes for honey:

- ✿ Antimicrobial
- ✿ Deodorisation
- ✿ Debriding
- ✿ Anti-inflammatory
- ✿ Stimulation of new tissue growth.

Currently, the literature on honey in wound care is mostly at case study level. This is useful in gaining a practical feel for what honey is capable of and, from an accountability point of view, the types of cases/situations in which it could be considered reasonable to use. But, this does not definitively inform us as to its value. There have been some clinical trials, but these studies are considered to be of low quality (Moore *et al*, 2001). As in most clinical situations, honey may not be the only active intervention being employed to effect a result, for example; antibiotics, pressure relief, bed rest and limb elevation, compression bandaging, and serial debridement may be being used simultaneously, thus making it difficult to determine outcomes attributable to honey. The clinical interest is aroused when these items have been recorded without the wound responding until the later addition of honey as a single additional measure.

Honey has a number of properties that could allow the reduction in the number of primary interface products on the shelf, making decision making in wound dressing choice far simpler (*Table 4.1*). So long as simple absorbent gauze and pads are available as backing dressings, a great many wounds can be treated. Provided that honey remains in contact with the wound and does not dilute and completely wash away before dressings are changed, then it is non-stick. It is also antimicrobial with no known resistance, aids debridement of necrotic tissue and slough, controls fluid through osmotic potential, and, in combination with alginate or simple backing dressings, prevents the maceration often seen with hydrogels and hydrocolloids. The main problem is that, in general, frequent dressing changes are needed, making it less convenient and challenging cost-effectiveness. Consideration needs to be given as to whether it is used in the short term, ie. to set a wound on the right track before transferring to products that will maintain the advantage, but be less time-consuming to administer. For example, honey would not be suitable under a four-layer compression bandage because of the infrequent changes associated with that bandaging.

The decision to employ a honey regime can be considered utilising the wound bed preparation/TIME concept and can be put into local dressing choice algorithms (*Figures 4.1* and *4.2*).

Table 4.1: Matching the dressing to the wound

Clinical activity/need	Current common use product	Honey alternative
Debridement: ❖ hard/leathery black or dark brown	Hydrogel	Liquid/gel honey*
❖ softening yellow brown eschar	Hydrogel sheet	Honey tulle*
❖ sloughy/wet	Hydrocolloid; hydrofibre; alginate	Honey alginate
Draining/cleaning sinuses	Capillary action absorbents	Liquid honey/honey soaked ribbon gauze or honey tulle strips
Cavity management	Alginates; hydrofibres; foams/hydropolymers	Honey alginate — using soft gauze to back fill larger cavities behind the primary honey dressing — small cavity/depressions managed with liquid/gel honey and occlusive film dressing
Critically colonised wounds	Silver and iodine products	Honey alginate or tulle
Infected wounds	Silver and iodine products with systemic antibiotics	Honey alginate or tulle with systemic antibiotics
Overgranulation	Topical steroid or steroid/antibiotic formulations; silver nitrate; silver and iodine dressings; local pressure; foams/hydropolymers	Honey tulle (does not require localisation to wound — it can overlap surrounding skin without causing maceration)
Indolence (no granulation; no edge advancement)	Protease inhibitors; silver or iodine products; sharp debridement	Honey tulle
Odour control	Metronidazole gel; silver products; charcoal products	Honey tulle or liquid honey — honey alginate might be useful in fungating breast wounds if the alginate maintains its haemostatic properties

* Caution may further dehydrate eschar preventing removal — although this may be a valuable feature in the ischaemic diabetic foot to prevent increase in size of lesions which can extend due to wet necrosis. It may also be a valuable effect prior to surgical debridement to demarcate the lesion and make it easier to grip and cut away (collaborate with the surgeon to find out if this is their preference).

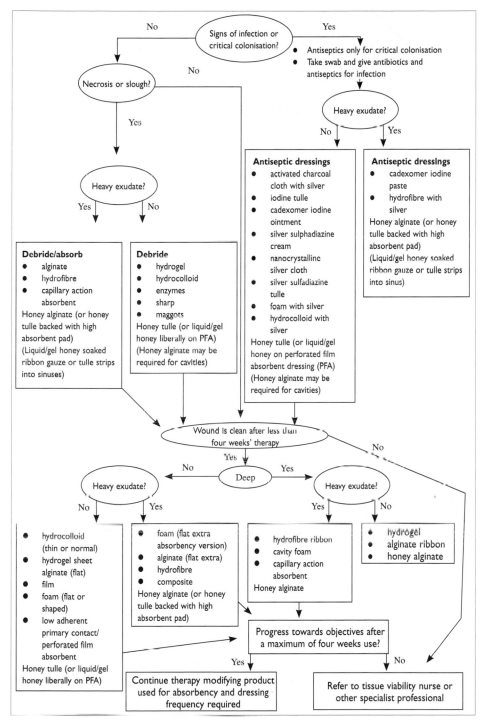

Figure 4.1: Primary dressing selection flow chart including honey

Clinical Observations	Proposed patho-physiology	WBP clinical actions	My trust/organisation nursing formulary choices	Effect of WBP actions
Tissue non-viable or deficient	Defective matrix and cell debris impair healing	Debridement (episodic or continuous) Autolytic, Sharp/surgical, Enzymatic, Mechanical, Biological	1st choice: hydrogel 2nd choice: l iquid/gel honey applied thickly onto suitable carrier, or occluded using a film dressing, or in a tulle or alginate ready to apply format. Dressing frequency dictated by the duration that honey remains in contact — probable change every 2 days when necrosis is dry, daily — twice daily when wound is autolysing and wet. Refer to TVN if no activity at 4 weeks' use. Expect result to be noticeable reduction of necrotic tissue within 2 weeks	Restoration of wound base and functional extra-cellular matrix proteins **(Viable wound base)**
Infection or inflammation	High bacterial counts or prolonged inflammation: ↑ Inflammatory cytokines ↑ Protease activity ↓ Growth factor activity	Remove infected foci using topical/systemic • antimicrobials • anti-inflammatories • protease inhibitors	**Wounds with cellulitis** 1st choice: antibiotics +/- antiseptic iodine or silver compound in formulation to suit moisture levels 2nd choice: honey in format to suit wound **Critically colonised wounds** 1st choice: antiseptic iodine or silver compound in formulation to suit moisture levels 2nd choice: honey in suitable format **Overgranulated wounds** 1st choice: honey tulle	Low bacterial counts or controlled inflammation: ↓ Inflammatory cytokines ↓ Protease activity ↑ Growth factor activity **(Bacterial balance and reduced inflammation)**
Moisture imbalance	Dessication slows epithelial cell migration Excessive fluid causes maceration of wound margin	Apply moisture balancing dressings Compression, negative pressure or other methods of removing fluid	**Macerated wounds** 1st choice: honey alginate (or honey tulle plus absorbent backing) to increase exudate absorption and bind water from saturated skin **High exudate wounds** 1st choices: alginate/hydrofibre or foam 2nd choice: honey alginate to reduce output via osmotic potential of honey **Dry wounds** 1st choice: hydrogel	Restored epithelial cell migration, dessication avoided, oedema, excessive fluid controlled, maceration avoided **(Moisture balanced)**
Epidermal margin, non-advancing or undermined	Non-migrating kertinocytes. Non-res-ponsive wound cells and abnormalities in extra-cellular matrix or protease activity	Reassess cause or consider corrective therapies: • debridement • skin grafts • biological agents • adjunctive therapies	**Recently 'stuck' wound** 1st choice: silver or iodine antiseptic dressing in formulation to suit moisture levels 2nd choice: honey in suitable format **Long-standing 'stuck' wound** 1st choice: honey in suitable format	Migrating keratinocytes and responsive wound cells. Restoration of appropriate protease profile. **(Advancing edge of wound)**

Figure 4.2: Local dressing choice

Case studies

The following section examines the various attributes listed above from a clinical case perspective.

Case study 1

Mr A — an eighty-year-old man with mixed arterial/venous ulcers on his right calf and medial malleolus. The ulcerations have occasionally shown signs of improvement, but never completely healed. On examination on 23 November 2004, the ulcers were indolent and considered critically colonised despite previous protease inhibitor (Promogran™, Johnson and Johnson) and cadexomer iodine (Iodoflex™, Smith and Nephew) use. Consequently, the treatment objectives were to debride, reduce bioburden and promote healing (see _Table 4.1_). Sharp debridement of the ulcer surface was undertaken and a calcification removed from the proximal ulcer bed. On review at 21 December 2004, honey tulle was applied to achieve the set treatment objectives. This was continued by the district nurse (_Figures 4.3_ and _4.4_).

Case study 2

Mr B — an eighty-year-old man with rheumatoid arthritis has had leg ulceration for two and a half years. He is fully mobile but has restricted ankle movement and fallen foot arches, and walks with a stiff leg gait. The ulcers are of venous aetiology. Compression bandaging was the mainstay of therapy. He is awaiting a hernia repair which is delayed due to presence of ulceration which increases the risk of infection should repair be performed whilst an ulcer is present. The treatment objectives were to heal the wound as quickly as possible to facilitate the planned surgery (_Figures 4.5_, _4.6_ and _4.7_).

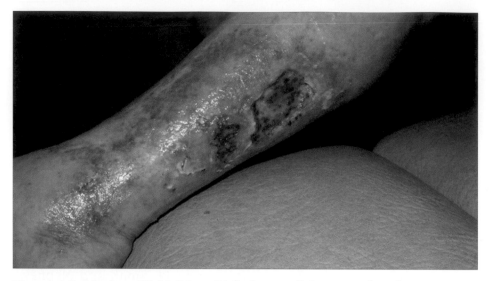

Figure 4.3: Mr A — 23.11.04 — Right leg medial aspect after sharp debridement and removal of a calcification from the proximal ulcer. Purulent exudate, some pain surrounding the ulcer but no obvious cellulitis. The ulcer is critically colonised and treatment continues with a protease inhibitor and cadexomer iodine. The glistening surface is just applied skin sealant (Cavilon cream™, 3M)

Case study 3

Mr C — was a forty-nine-year-old man with a twenty-five-year history of painful venous ulceration refractory to vein surgery and compression bandaging. He was hospitalised in 2000 for topical wound care of these painful, sloughy, malodorous, highly exuding ulcers, with associated varicose eczema. Initial debridement was undertaken using maggots (Kingsley, 2001). Honey dressings were applied to address the need for debridement, control of malodour, and reduction of exudate attributed to high bioburden.

Case study 4

Mr D — a seventy-six-year-old man with a history of mixed arterial and venous disease had stopped going to bed at night due to ischaemic pain. His right leg was chronically swollen and very wet, which was the reason why he would not return to bed. Exposed swollen tendon was present and covered with soft yellow slough. Mr D had arterial bypass surgery in late 2004 but Doppler ABPI remained low at 0.67 (left = 0.54). To improve the wound it is necessary to reduce swelling which might best be effected by elevation, given that poor arterial supply rules out continuous compression bandaging. Going to bed at night was only possible if full containment of exudates was achieved, as current bandages, however well padded, become wet through within a few hours (*Figure 4.8*).

Case study 5

Ms E — a young woman with a seemingly spontaneous abscess eruption on her left cheek, which was neither tooth infection or of trauma origin. She was given antibiotics and the abscess was drained by a maxillo-facial surgeon. The lump started rising again a few days after with slightly haemorrhagic colouration but without tenderness or exudation (*Figure 4.9*).

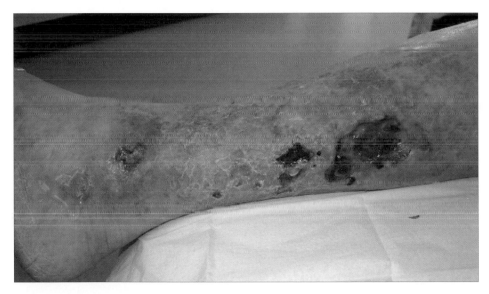

Figure 4.4: Mr A — 21.12.04 — Right leg medial aspect mixed aetiology ulceration. Distal ulcer is infected (painful, erythematous and enlarged) despite use of cadexomer iodine, antiobiotics have been prescribed. Other ulcers remain critically colonised (static). Honey tulle application to start today

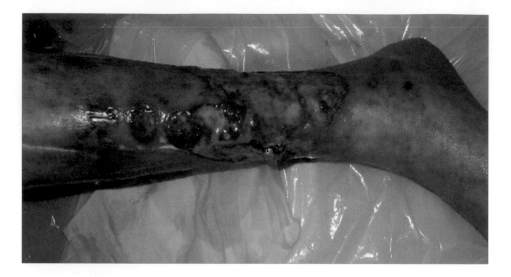

Figure 4.5: Mr B — 18.11.04 — Right leg medial aspect venous ulcer after ten days treatment with SSD cream and systemic antibiotics

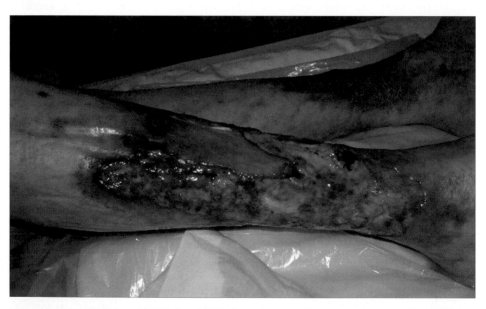

Figure 4.6: Mr B — 18.11.04 — Right leg lateral aspect venous ulcer after ten days treatment with SSD cream and systemic antibiotics

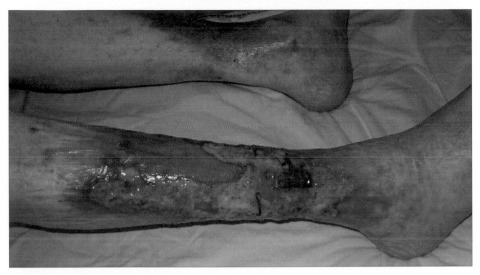

Figure 4.7: Mr B — 26.11.04 — Right leg lateral aspect venous ulcer after eighteen days treatment with SSD cream and systemic antibiotics

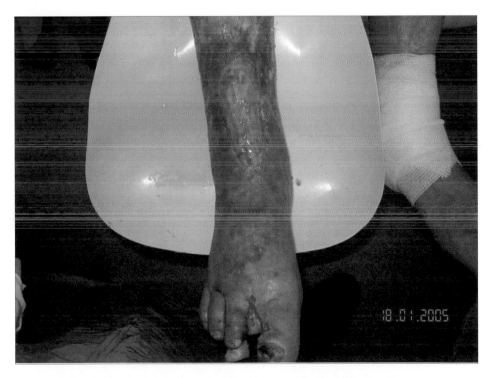

Figure 4.8: Mr D — 18.1.05 — Right leg mixed ulcer for treatment with honey tulle and Kerraboot to reduce swelling, control exudate and deslough ulcer surface

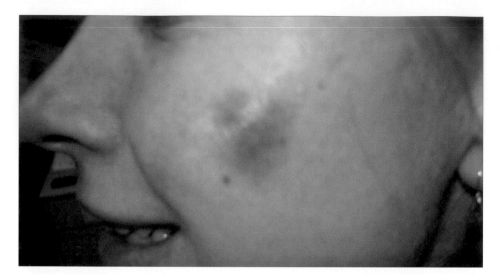

Figure 4.9: Ms E — 12.1.05 — Recent facial abscess site, following drainage and use of systemic antibiotics, a non-painful lump is appearing

Case study 6

Mrs F — a sixty-seven-year-old, fully mobile woman was admitted to a community hospital with painful infected ulcers. The ulcers had been static for some time and, despite antibiotic therapy, had continued to be painful although lessened. The left leg had suffered recurrent ulcerations and the patient had had phlebitis, eczema, ankle flare, dry skin and past venous surgery. The right leg ulcerated recently following traumatic injury from a bicycle accident in September 2004. The left medial ulcer presents in a stained atrophie blanche area posterior to the malleolus covered with a fibrinous slough and was considered critically colonised at the time of honey tulle application. A larger left lateral malleolus ulcer was considered borderline critically colonised/locally infected due to pain description by the patient and was also treated with honey tulle. In addition, a right medial ulcer was also concurrent and there were obvious varicosities on both legs. Further vein surgery was scheduled for March 2005. The right leg was treated with a silver hydrofibre dressing and weekly four-layer compression bandaging. The left leg was not compression bandaged due to ulcer pain. See *Figures 4.10* and *4.11*.

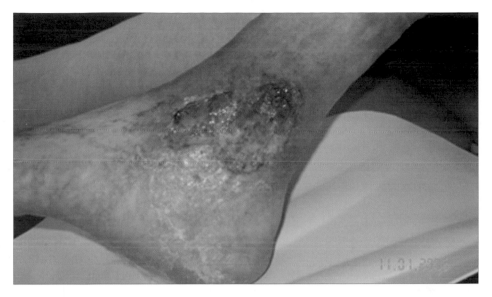

Figure 4.10: Mrs F — 11.1.05 — Left lateral malleolar venous ulcer prior to initial application of honey tulle

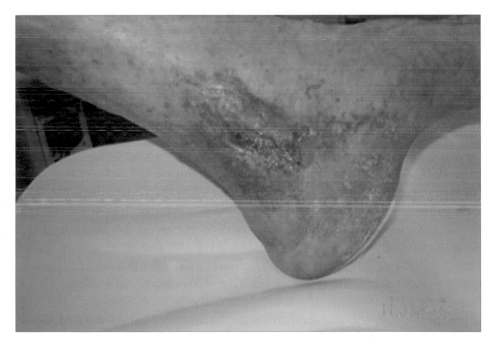

Figure 4.11: Mrs F — 11.1.5 — Left medial malleolar venous ulcer, indolent painful ulcer recently treated for infection by hospital admission, antibiotics and bed rest. Photo taken prior to initial application of honey tulle

20%. There was no obvious improvement to the left lateral ulcer (+1% surface area in four weeks) either. Despite honey, the left lateral ulcer has since become infected again, it is painful and stings for at least one hour after honey tulle application and gives discomfort all day of the dressing change. Honey therapy to ulcers has been stopped, antibiotics and silver foam dressings have been instituted to combat infection and reduce pain from honey application. Prevention of recurrent infection in the left lateral and improvement of the critical colonisation in the left medial in two weeks of therapy did not, in this case, occur in the ulcers to which honey was applied (*Figures 4.14* and *4.15*).

Deodorisation

Mr C — was keen to try honey on his ulcers after seeing a television programme. It was agreed to source a UMF10 liquid Manuka medical grade honey (Active 10+ Manuka Honey® from Comvita). Complete deodorisation was noted at the first dressing change at twenty-four hours — something which had not been achieved for him with other antiseptic dressings up to that date.

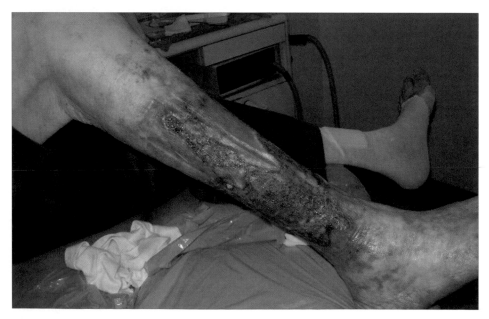

Figure 4.13: Mr B — 21.12.04 Right leg lateral aspect after fourteen days treatment with honey tulle

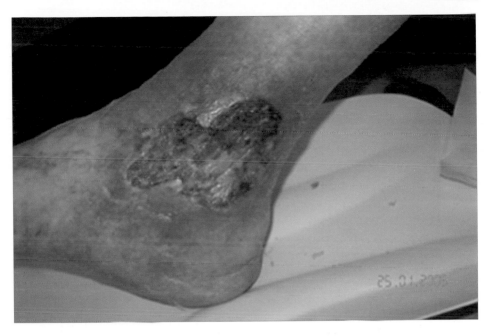

Figure 4.14: Mrs F — 25.1.05 — Left lateral malleolar venous ulcer diagnosed as infected from patient description of pain, continuing redness and darkening of ulcer tissue

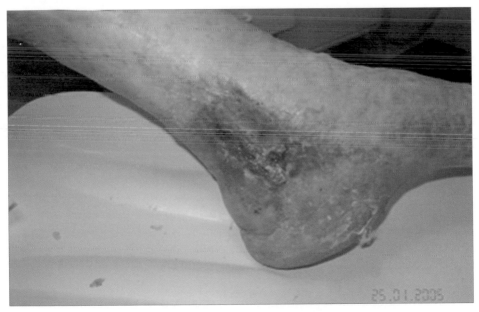

Figure 4.15: Mrs F — 25.1.05 — Left medial malleolar venous ulcer demonstrating an increase in size, despite fourteen-day use of honey tulle

Debriding

Mr D — after consulting with the tissue viability nurse, Mr D agreed to try a regime using Kerraboot® (Ark Therapeutics) to contain exudate at night so that he could return to bed rather than sleeping in the chair. Honey tulle was applied to effect debridement of the soft slough covering the wounds, notably the tendon. In addition, it was placed to aid control of exudate production by exerting osmotic control and reduce maceration present around the wounds. Despite encouragement, Mr D did not utilise the Kerraboot or return to sleeping in bed at night. The honey tulle increased his pain but did act to remove slough. A reasonably high elevation whilst sitting and sleeping in his chair did appear to reduce the generalised leg swelling, though the tendon remains proud (*Figure 4.8*).

Anti-inflammatory

Mr B — concurrent with the ulceration on the right leg, there remained a static ulcer on the left which had been treated with protease inhibitor under activated charcoal silver (Actisorb Silver™, Johnson and Johnson) and compression bandaging. From admission, the wound was clean but overgranulated. It had remained static despite the systemic antibiotic regime of the first three weeks of hospitalisation. Honey was initiated and healing took three weeks (in the continued presence of antibiotics, bed rest and without compression) (*Figures 4.16a, b, c*).

Ms E — honey was applied to the facial lump which arose following the drainage of the abscess to see if it would reduce the lump. It has been reported anecdotally that rising boils can be 'cured' by application (personal communication, P Molan, Harrogate Wounds UK conference 2004). After three applications, each less than twenty-four hours, Ms E reported that the lump had reduced in size. Following discussion with the TVN, she decided to try some further applications to see if it would reduce further. These facial dresssings were applied overnight to avoid potential embarrassment of wearing the dressing during the day (*Figure 4.17*).

Two recent anecdotal reports have been received of the significant effect on teenage facial acne within five days of overnight treament with

Manuka honey (UMF 18+). The correspondent noted, 'it changed my daughter's life' (practice nurse, R Poile, personal communication, March 2005).

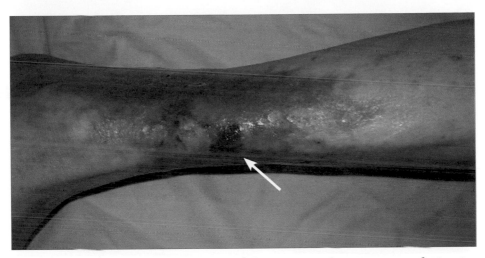

Figure 4.16a: Mr B — 26.11.04 — Left leg venous ulcer, overgranulation in clean but static left ulcer since admission on 18.11.05

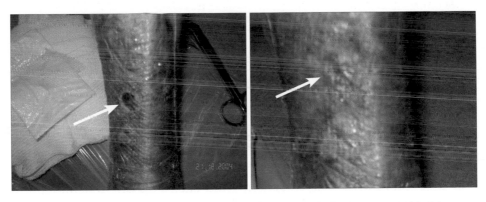

Figure 4.16b: Mr B — 21.12.04 — Left leg previously overgranulated venous ulcer, pre-crust removal

Figure 4.16c: Mr B — 21.12.04 — Left leg previously overgranulated venous ulcer, post-crust removal, healed wound

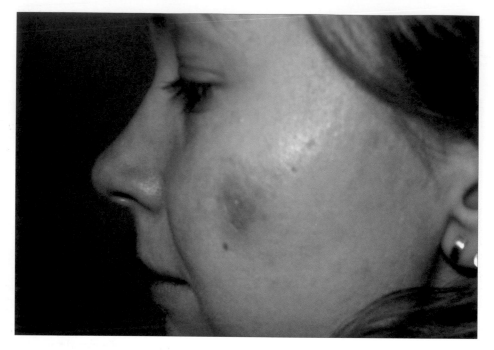

Figure 4.17: Ms E — 19.1.05 — Recent facial abscess site following three applications, each for less than twenty-four hours of honey tulle under simple paper island dressing. Patient reports swelling reduced. There were no other concurrent treatments

Stimulation of new tissue growth

Mr A — needed control of critical colonisation and also stimulation of new tissue, a difficult task considering the backdrop of ischaemia in the affected limb. Clinic review on 25 January 2005 showed an improvement through a reduction in surface area of 23.6% in four weeks of use, and full epithelialisation of a small <1cm² ulcer in the calf cluster (*Figures 4.18, 4.19, 4.20* and *4.21*).

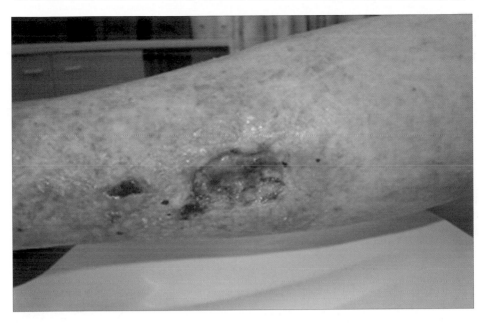

Figure 4.18: Mr A — 25.1.05 — Right leg medial aspect mixed aetiology ulcers, showing 23.6% area reduction after approximately four weeks use of honey tulle

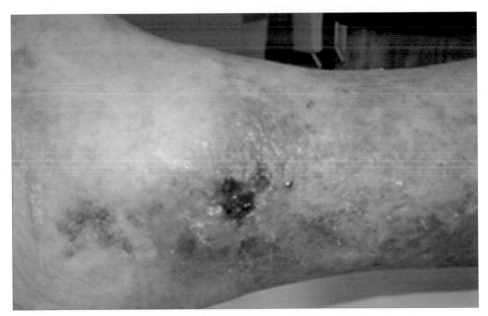

Figure 4.19: Mr A — 25.1.05 — Right leg medial malleolar ulcer improving under the influence of honey

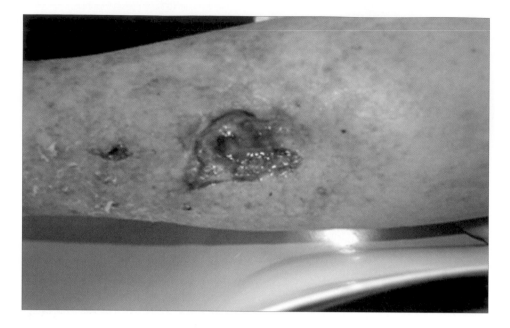

Figure 4.20: Mr A — 22.2.05 — Right leg medial aspect mixed aetiology ulcer cluster continuing to heal under the influence of honey

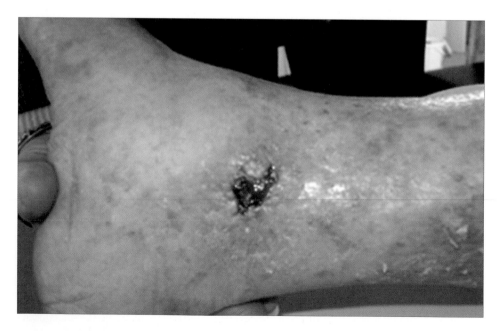

Figure 4.21: Mr A — 22.2.05 — Right leg medial malleolar ulcer continuing to improve under the influence of honey

Clinical outcomes

The outcome to measure the intervention with honey depends on the objective set when constructing a care plan. Firstly, it is necessary to set an overall goal of care, either to heal a wound and restore full function; or secondly, to alleviate symptoms. Controlling symptoms will also be necessary when progressing towards healing. Taking the healing goal first, the objective for the intervention will also depend on where the wound currently fits in the Wound Healing Continuum (Gray *et al*, 2004), and, whether there is any wound bed preparation to undertake before the wound can actually start to heal. For example, if a wound is covered with soft necrotic eschar, the objective would be to remove that within a certain length of time. This time period should be the time you would expect your usual therapy, such as a hydrogel, to achieve this on a patient in the same condition, such as three weeks. At the end of that period, the objective is posed as a question, 'Was all the necrotic tissue removed as planned in three weeks?', the answer being yes or no. In addition, you can also determine how much faster or slower than expected the intervention took. Over time, the use of this simple technique will give the practitioner a good idea of the value of the intervention, whether it is better, same, or worse than the usual therapy. Outcomes can be plotted and documented using the Applied Wound Management system (Gray *et al*, 2004), which uses three continuums to monitor key features in the wound: tissue colour, infection and exudate. The system will soon be widely available as software and in paper formats, perhaps for the first time supporting the routine gathering of clear outcome data in the UK to demonstrate efficacy of interventions. Outside specialist centres in the UK, outcome monitoring has been rarely undertaken routinely, with practitioners focusing more on the journey quality rather than the speed to the final destination: so, establishing efficacy of honey over other regimes in general clinical practice is presently likely to be anecdotal at best.

Once the wound is prepared, outcomes, in terms of size reduction, can be undertaken most simply by serial recording of maximum length and breadth, or by using simple tracing on squared acetate transparencies. A digital planimetry system is now widely available called Visitrak® (Smith and Nephew) that combines the acetate with automatic calculation of surface area, allowing repeat tracings to demonstrate surface area reduction over time. It is easy to use and within the budget of many clinical teams who only need one unit to share between team members (for example, all district and practice nurses at a surgery, as the tracing of the wound can be brought back to base for calculation on the Visitrak®). Flanagan (2003) stated in a literature review that healing wounds should reduce by over 40% surface area in two to three weeks. Clinical experience would suggest that this measure of time should begin as soon as the wound bed is prepared; that is, cleared of any initial presenting necrotic tissue and control of infection. Anything less than 20% in the two- to three-week period following initial wound bed preparation, shows that the wound is not responding. Measurement linked to time is crucial to evaluation of wound care interventions.

Instead of healing outcomes, symptom control can be monitored in a variety of ways. For example, if the objective of using a honey product is to unblock a critical colonisation, as evidenced by the blue green staining produced by *Pseudomonas aeruginosa* seen on dressings, then the timepoint at which to measure the outcome and, therefore, the effectiveness of the product is short. A result for a topical antimicrobial strategy should be short, eg. seven days. If any antimicrobial intervention takes longer to achieve the desired outcome, the wound may have enlarged in the meantime suggesting that the intervention is either not effective or not optimal. Pain control using a visual analogue scale or one to ten point scale could be undertaken at dressing change to gauge background, breakthrough and procedural pain to determine if trends are in the appropriate direction. Honey does have a tendency to sting, probably due to its acidic pH, for up to an hour after application, so the use of analgesia pre-application is often necessary. Odour control could be monitored using TELER (Browne *et al*, 2004) type statements, such as odour experienced on entry to house, on entry to the bedroom, when at bedside, or on removal of dressing, allowing a quantification of sorts of odour experienced. Depending on what the level of experience was at the outset of the intervention, a patient negotiated outcome point could be worked towards, such as absence of odour until dressing is removed. Odour can contribute to social isolation and nausea leading to poor nutrition so the time to outcome is important. Honey might be expected to make an impact on long-standing odour problems in seven days, any later would indicate lack of efficacy.

Conclusion

The use of modern honey products shows clinical promise for the wound care practitioner. The honey in the 'Medical Devices' seems to be an excellent and rapid deodoriser. Quick resolution of this unpleasant occurrence may aid concordance with the whole wound care regime. Correction of overgranulation seems to suggest it is directly anti-inflammatory, or indirectly so through an antimicrobial action, and, in the case study described, facilitated epithelialisation (*p. 72*). Whether this effect resulted from stimulation of cells to divide, or removal of hindrance to healing, is not known. The reduction of the facial swelling below unbroken skin would suggest that an active component penetrates the epidermis. This is particularly interesting as there is little evidence to demonstrate that conventional antiseptics penetrate into the interstitium and act below wound beds, where invasive pathogens cause damage, let alone enter through intact skin. However, it is known that silver and iodine can be found at sites in the body remote to the wound, demonstrating systemic absorption from open wounds. In addition to the benefits listed by Molan, there may be benefit in the direction of healing without scarring which has been touched on by Topham (2002) and Lusby *et al* (2002).

There are two principal downsides of honey. Firstly, it often stings on application, though this can be ameliorated by pre-procedural analgesia and tolerated by the patient if they are prepared in advance to expect this for a limited time. Secondly, honey requires frequent reapplication, often once or twice daily at the start of a regime and, from experience, does not last longer than three days. It should also be remembered that not all honeys have the same activity: careful selection of a medical grade product is necessary. Honey has certainly started to capture the imagination of patients, practitioners and dressing manufacturers but, whether it gains full acceptance as a routine, rather than as a specialist product, remains to be seen.

References

Browne N, Grocott P, Cowley S *et al* (2004) Woundcare Research for Appropriate Products (WRAP); validation of the TELER method. *Int J Nurs Stud* **41**(5): 559–71

Flanagan M (2003) Wound measurement: can it help us to monitor progression to healing? *J Wound Care* **12**(5): 189–94

Gray D, White R, Cooper C, Kingsley A (2004) The wound healing continuum, an aid to clinical decision making and clinical audit. *Applied Wound Management Supplement*. Wounds-UK. www.wounds-uk.com: 9–12

Kingsley A (2001) The use of honey in the treatment of infected wounds: case studies. *Br J Nursing* **10**(22) Tissue Viability Supplement: s13–s20

Lusby P, Coombes A, Wilkinson J (2002) Honey: A potent agent for wound healing. *J Wound Ostomy Continence Nurs* **29**(6): 295–99

Molan P (1999) The role of honey in the management of wounds. *J Wound Care* **8**(8): 415–18

Moore O, Smith L, Campbell F, Seers K, McQuay H, Moore R (2001) Systematic review of the use of honey as a wound dressing. *BMC Complementary and Alternative Medicine* **1**(2) www.biomedcentral.com/1472-6882/1/2

Topham J (2002) Why do some cavity wounds treated with honey or sugar paste heal without scarring? *J Wound Care* **11**(2): 53–5

CHAPTER 5

THE USE OF LEPTOSPERMUM HONEY IN CHRONIC WOUND MANAGEMENT

Val Robson

In recent years the use of honey to manage wounds has gained considerable interest. One outcome of this has been the commercial development of regulated 'medical quality' honey and honey-based dressings. The clinical evidence for honey in wound care is reviewed in *Chapter 9*. To complement this review, and to add the patient perspectives, a selection of case studies is presented. The aim being to offer practical advice for the choice of honey, practical aspects of wound treatment, and, clinical outcomes. The following cases demonstrate the 'multifunctional' properties of one commercially available honey: control of bioburden, reduction of inflammation, skin care, and, exudate management.

Case study 1

Mrs C developed venous leg ulceration due to venous hypertension. The ulcer was initially treated with compression bandage therapy. However, after twelve weeks the wound had failed to heal so the patient was referred for vascular opinion. A colour duplex Doppler ultrasound scan revealed gross short saphenous vein (SSV) reflux. Ligation and avulsion of the SSV was performed to assist healing of the ulcer. The patient was reviewed as an outpatient four weeks later, but, despite surgery, the ulcer persisted. A wound swab taken during surgery confirmed the presence of *Staphylococcus aureus*, *Pseudomonas spp* and Haemolytic Streptococcus (Group B). The patient was commenced on ciprofloxacin 500 mgs bd for seven days.

Four months after surgery, the patient was becoming very frustrated as the ulcer still refused to heal and was affecting her quality of life. In an attempt to resolve the problem, Mrs C was admitted to hospital for split skin grafting and excision of the ulcer, as it was considered that grafting may offer the best chance of healing. During the procedure three biopsies of tissue were removed and sent for histology, which confirmed extensive epidermal ulceration and dense inflammation. The dermis was infiltrated by a well-differentiated invasive squamous cell carcinoma.

The patient was discharged after seven weeks. The skin graft had taken well but the donor site was over-granulating — this was being treated with a topical steroid. Mrs C was reviewed in clinic on a regular basis; at nine months the graft site had healed but the donor site had not.

The patient was referred to the wound care clinic. At this stage she was exasperated that the original area of ulceration which had been skin grafted had healed but she now had four areas of superficial skin loss causing similar problems to the original wound. She found bandages uncomfortable, they often slipped, causing damage to the delicate granulation tissue, and dressings used to manage exudate adhered to the wound — and were, therefore, painful to remove.

The four areas contained some over-granulation, indicative of prolonged inflammation, there was moderate exudate, and the surrounding area was normal. Mrs C was experiencing a moderate amount of pain. The analgesia prescribed by her GP was controlling this satisfactorily. A wound swab confirmed the presence of mixed skin flora (*Figure 5.1*).

As a possible remedy, it was felt that the use of topical honey would provide a protective barrier whilst treating the overgranulation, consequently reducing the exudate and pain Mrs C was experiencing. Having managed the wound itself the surrounding area of skin was treated with Cavilon™ barrier spray (3M Ltd) with an adhesive foam dressing applied to contain the honey. Initially, the community nursing service renewed the dressing three times per week (*Figure 5.2*).

At review two weeks later the area was healing, and the exudate and pain had reduced. The dressing regime was continued as before, but at this stage Mrs C was able to manage the dressing herself twice weekly (*Figure 5.3*).

Four weeks after the commencement of honey treatment the wound had healed. Mrs C was advised to keep the area moisturised to protect the skin and also prevent friction injury.

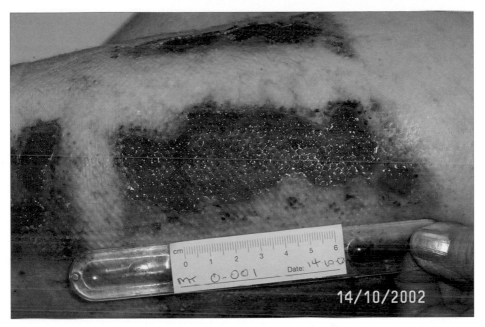

Figure 5.1: Case 1 — The donor site showing signs of overgranulation. The area was painful, moderately exuding, and dressing adherence was a problem. A wound swab showed mixed skin flora

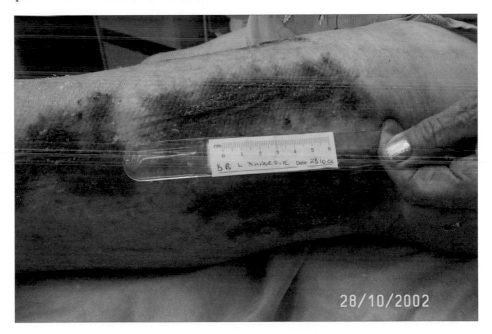

Figure 5.2: Case 1 — Following application of honey under an adhesive foam dressing for two weeks, the area showed positive signs of healing

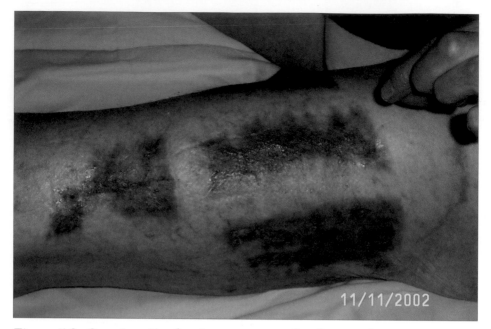

11/11/2002

Figure 5.3: Case 1 — Further improvement after four weeks' treatment with the with honey dressing. Re-epithelialisation evident

Case study 2

Mr D is a sixty-year-old gentleman. He is mobile and self-caring. In March 2001, Mr D had pantalar fusion of his left ankle following a fracture. However, in January 2002 Mr D was admitted for the removal of the metal work and incision and drainage of an abscess in the left ankle region. Treatment included a period of bed rest and elevation and intravenous antibiotic therapy. On review in clinic two months following admission, the wounds appeared clean and healthy and a further course of antibiotics was prescribed.

After nine months, Mr D's wounds had still failed to heal. He was referred to a consultant plastic surgeon with a view to split skin grafting to the wounds on the lateral and medial malleoli. The wounds were reported to be granulating but recalcitrant. On examination by the plastic surgeon, Mr D's left ankle was red and swollen and had a 2 cm deep open wound, discharging pus. An x-ray was performed which did not show any evidence of osteomyelitis and the wound swabs confirmed *Staphylococcus aureus* and anaerobes, sensitive to flucloxacillin and metronidazole.

The plastic surgeon considered Mr D to have underlying peripheral vascular disease and, therefore, referred him for vascular opinion.

On examination by the vascular surgeon, Mr D had no palpable pedal pulses but had palpable femoral and popliteal pulses and good Doppler signals in the proximal anterior tibial and posterior tibial arteries.

Mr D was referred to the wound clinic in April 2003. The ulcers on the medial and lateral malleoli had a small amount of slough present within the wound. The surrounding areas were red and dry with no heat or swelling (*Figures 5.4a* and *5.4b*).

Despite a plethora of dressings and the best efforts of the community nurses, the wounds refused to heal.

Mr D was advised to shower or bathe prior to wound dressing to assist with removal of dry skin, and to aid re-hydration of the dry skin around the wounds. Honey was applied to the ulceration and honey mixed with an emollient to the surrounding area two to three times per week. The honey was applied to a non-adherent dressing at approximately 3 mm depth, with a surgipad and wool and crepe bandage to secure.

At review in four weeks, the surrounding redness was starting to settle and there had been some debridement of slough within the wounds (*Figures 5.5a, 5.5b*).

At twenty-four weeks, Mr D's ulcer had almost healed and was about the size of a pinhead, there was no exudate and no pain. The redness surrounding the ulceration had completely disappeared. He was continuing to apply honey to the wound.

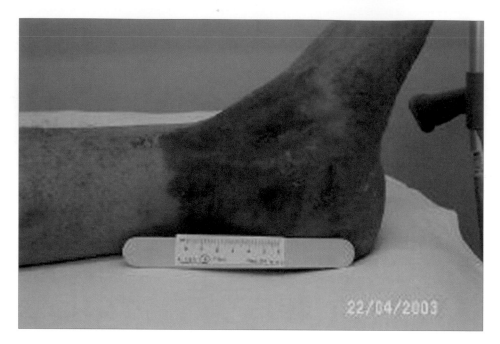

Figure 5.4a: Case 2 — Medial ulcer at start of honey treatment. This wound had been present for nine months; note the extensive inflammation

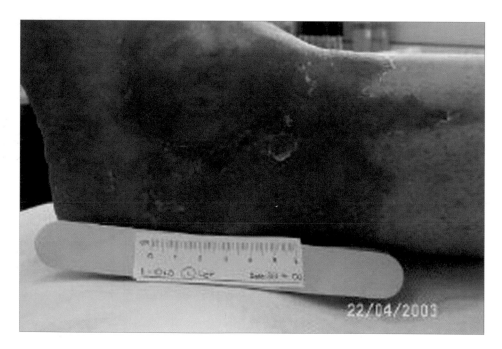

Figure 5.4b: Case 2 — Lateral ulcer also showing extensive erythema

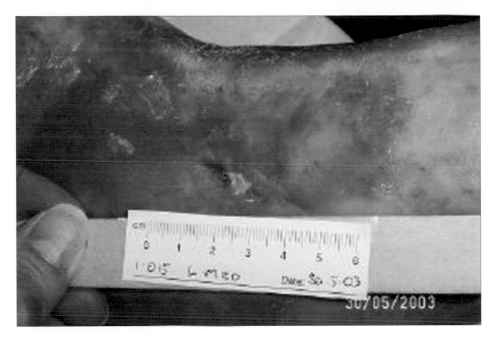

Figure 5.5a: Case 2 — Medial ulcer after six weeks' treatment with honey. The erythema is reduced and discharge minimal

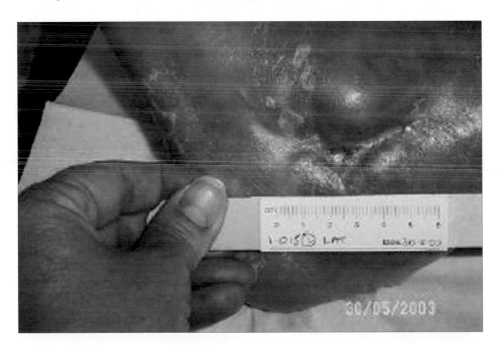

Figure 5.5b: Case 2 — Lateral ulcer also showing positive signs of healing

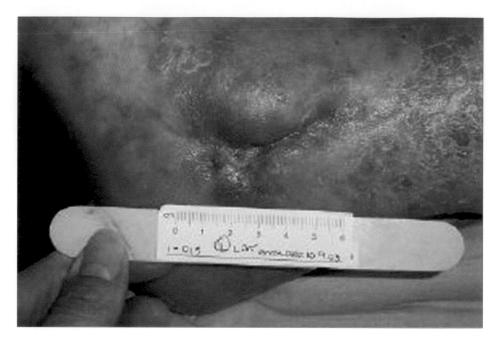

Figure 5.6: Case 2 — Lateral ulcer, September 2003

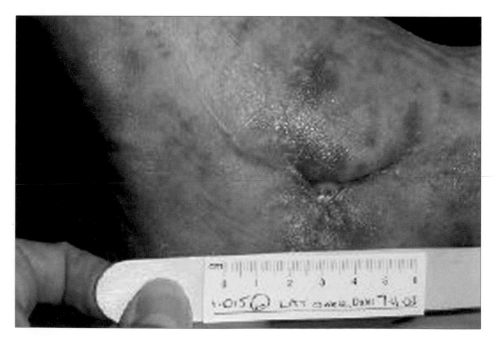

Figure 5.7a: Case 2 — The lateral ulcer almost healed

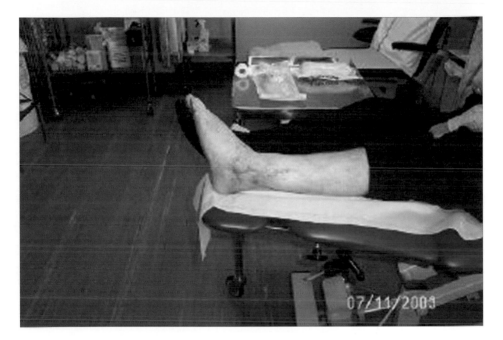

Figure 5.7b: Case 2 — The lateral ulcer at the point of closure. Inflammation greatly reduced

Discussion

In both these cases the wounds appeared to be stranded in the inflammatory phase of healing. In normal wound healing the inflammatory stage lasts for approximately three days but may be prolonged. When this happens a chronic inflammatory stage is established and the wound does not move on into the proliferation stage of healing.

Honey has a direct anti-inflammatory effect on wounds, not a secondary effect from the antibacterial action removing the bacteria that cause inflammation. Honey applied to the wounds and surrounding area resolved the inflammatory effect of the wound allowing it to progress.

Acknowledgements

The honey used in all the case studies is MediHoney™ presented in 30g tubes that had been gamma irradiated without affecting the antibacterial activity. MediHoney™ is produced in Australia by Medihoney Pty Ltd and is a standardised mix of antibacterial honeys including Australian and New Zealand *Leptospermum spp*.

Data for all these case studies is collected using the Leg Ulcer Telemedicine Medicine System (LUTMS), designed by Good Hope Hospital, West Midlands. LUTMS is a dedicated, secure, shared electronic patient record. The LUTMS has been designed to allow the incorporation of colour digital images in the electronic patient record. The LUTMS includes ulcer size measurement and automatically plots ulcer-healing rate. Information regarding the LUTMS can be obtained by contacting simon.dodds@goodhope.nhs.uk

Support

University Hospital Aintree
University Hospital Aintree Research Committee
The Florence Nightingale Foundation
The Florence Nightingale Council
The Huntleigh Foundation
MediHoney Pty Ltd, Australia

CHAPTER 6

QUALITY STANDARDS OF MEDICAL GRADE MANUKA HONEY

Young Mee Yoon and Claire Newlands

The concept of 'medical grade honey' started in August 2000 following global demand for high quality medical grade honey and honey-based health products. Our company, Comvita, specifically its medical division, has ongoing activities in honey research and intellectual property development together with the University of Waikato, Hamilton, New Zealand. The company currently holds a range of honey product patents and also participates and funds numerous research and clinical trials for further product development and extension. The research interest of the company extends from wound care to oral/dental hygiene, throat care, internal health, skin care, eye care and immune support.

A unique accredited honey supply programme has been developed as company intellectual property to meet the quality requirements of Medical Device manufacturing internationally. The programme includes an accredited supplier network with the development of quality standards and systems for honey resourcing, harvesting and extraction. Quality management standards and systems have also been developed for honey processing. Strict product testing regimes were also set for ensuring the integrity of 'medical grade honey' supply.

Whilst some of the more exact components of the medical grade honey processing and measuring techniques, as well as the supply programme, are held confidentially within intellectual property management, this chapter gives an overview of the exacting efforts put in to ensure that the honey used in the medical arena is of true 'medical grade'.

The systems developed for the programme were done in consideration of preventing any possible microbiological, physical and chemical contamination that cannot be removed afterwards, and also for the prevention of natural quality deterioration/loss during storage. Traceability of the honey from hive to finished product is also an essential part of the system developed. A series of workshops with landowners, beekeepers and honey extractors have been carried out to introduce the concept of 'medical grade honey', and to develop standards and systems. At the end of the supply programme an assessment is undertaken of the suppliers, and only the suppliers that pass the assessment are able to supply medical grade honey. The accredited suppliers are also regularly audited and monitored by Comvita, throughout each honey season, to ensure compliance with the standards and systems developed.

We are committed to improving continually the quality of medical grade honey by conducting full breakdown analysis on resource sites, harvesting/beekeeper practices and extraction processes, including a full analysis of all inward raw medical grade honey received each season. Supplier management manuals are updated annually as improvements are required. Feedback and improvement meetings with suppliers are held regularly to ensure that all supplier practices are kept up-to-date and current.

Introduction

The use of honey as a topical antibacterial agent has been emphasised by New Zealand's University of Waikato Professor, Dr Peter Molan, since 1989, and is gaining acceptance for the treatment of surface infections such as ulcers, burns, injuries, pressure ulcers, and surgical wounds (Cooper *et al*, 2001; Cooper and Molan, 1999; Molan, 1998; Molan, 2001). A feature of the usage of active Manuka honey is the rapid clearance of infection, in many cases from wounds that had not responded to various forms of conventional treatment (Cooper *et al*, 1999; Molan and Allen, 1996).

The supply programme is a unique framework of partnership in land use and honey supply, working together with landowners and beekeepers, to ensure continuing and expanding economic benefit from premium quality medical grade Manuka honey. It was developed from an unwavering commitment to sustainable resource management and robustness of medical grade honey supply into the Medical Device market. The concept started in August 2000 following global interest in, and demand for, high quality medical grade honey and honey-based health products. Through the consumer and specialty product activities, the company seeks to introduce therapeutic and beneficial effects of honey to all those with a concern for natural health.

We are continuing to develop close business relationships with international companies involved in relevant clinical, therapeutic and health-related products for development, distribution and manufacturing of Medical Device/therapeutic honey products.

Microbiological quality control for medical grade honey

There is a risk of introducing micro-organisms into wounds, especially botulism, if honey is used as a dressing (Molan and Allen, 1996). The risk can be avoided by sterilisation. Gamma irradiation is one of the more common sterilisation methods in the wound dressing industry and it was found that gamma irradiation does not affect the antibacterial activity of honey (Molan and Allen, 1996). An international Medical Device ingredient microbiological requirement for manufacturing is a total plate count (TPC) of less than 500 colony forming units (cfu) per gram (g). The microbiological specification is required to meet a pre-sterilisation (gamma irradiation) requirement, ensuring the sterilisation process is always successful; thereby eliminating the risk of introducing micro-organisms into wounds from honey dressings.

Primary microbiological contamination sources for honey include pollen, the digestive tracts of honey bees, dust, air, earth and nectar. The secondary contamination sources (processing, after harvest) include air, water, human/honey handlers, honey extraction and processing equipment and buildings (Snowdon, 1999; Snowdon and Cliver, 1996). Due to the natural physical properties of honey that serve to inhibit microbial growth — ie. low moisture (less than 21%), low water activity (A_w 0.5–0.6) and acidic environment (pH 3.4–6.1), the microbes of concern are from contamination; especially from post-harvest handling (Snowdon and Cliver, 1996).

Commonly found microbes in honey are osmophilic or sugar tolerant yeasts, moulds and spore-forming bacteria. Our medical grade honey processing system has been validated to ensure any existing yeast and mould cells, if present, are destroyed effectively, without damaging any honey quality aspects. However, removal of contaminated spore-forming bacteria (eg. from the genus *Bacillus*) in honey is not easy; the bacterial load does not reduce during storage, unlike other certain vegetative cells that have been known to decrease after time in honey, due to its antimicrobial properties that discourage the growth or persistence of many micro-organisms (Snowdon and Cliver, 1996). The honey supply programme, which is being managed very successfully, focuses on the prevention of possible spore-forming bacterial contamination.

Due to strict hygiene control from honey collection to honey extracting and processing, possible contamination of micro-organisms (eg. coliform bacteria and pathogenic bacteria such as *Staphylococcus*, *Salmonella* and *Clostridium* species) that indicate poor sanitary quality of honey has not been an issue for the medical grade honey supply programme. Strict packaging standards and storage conditions for extracted honey have also helped in the prevention of possible microbial increases during storage.

Development and management of a honey supply programme

Historically, the microbiological total plate count level of honey could vary from less than 100 cfu/g to greater than 50000 cfu/g. From this historical information on the variance of microbiological levels in honey, the need was recognised to develop a supplier programme to control possible microbiological contamination during the harvesting, extraction and processing stages of honey collection. Adding to the international Medical Device ingredient requirements are specifications for physical and chemical contamination, as well as accurate and reliable traceability of the honey from hive to finished product. These additional factors only reconfirmed the need for a robust mechanism for sustainable medical grade honey supply into the international Medical Device market.

To meet the Medical Device ingredient requirements, a supplier network was developed, with suppliers accredited to our organisation ensuring compliance of quality standards and systems. These standards and systems have been developed with the suppliers, to ensure adequacy and practicability of implementation from the Manuka resources to honey harvesting and extraction, and also for honey processing. The strict raw material and finished product specifications for Medical Device ingredients are adhered to rigorously to ensure that honey supplied to the international market is of appropriate quality.

Overview

Operating at the heart of the supply and production chain, we have established quality management polices and procedures, setting and ensuring maximum achievable standards to cover the total resource management, product sourcing, harvest, extraction and production cycle. Throughout, we operate to and demand stringent and comprehensive risk management and conformance policies.

Figure 6.1 shows the integrated supply chain management for the extended honey supply programme, which was implemented in 2002, and has been operating effectively ever since.

The honey supply programme involved a series of workshops and education days with landowners, beekeepers and honey extractors. The purpose was to introduce the concept of 'medical grade honey' and develop standards and systems that would enable stringent quality specifications to be met. Once the concept of medical grade honey was introduced to the suppliers, draft protocols for quality management standards were developed and reviewed for each stage of the raw material honey supply chain. Once reviewed, a final set of standards were developed and issued for implementation. Prior to final implementation in the field, one of the last parts of the programme included an assessment of the quality standards. Only those suppliers that pass the assessment are able to supply raw medical grade honey for analysis.

We now have a considerable number of contracted accredited medical grade honey suppliers and extractors, as well as a large pool of contracted general honey suppliers with the potential to become accredited medical grade honey suppliers, as and when honey dressing product growth is seen in the market. We are committed to ensuring large stock piles of medical grade honey are kept available to respond to any market growth for honey dressing products.

Medical grade Manuka honey is grown from a specific resource and harvested and processed purely for that purpose. The Manuka plant is a rapid growing, hardy plant and is native to New Zealand. The Manuka resource of New Zealand is in plentiful supply, which has by no means been exhausted; again allowing for potential future growth of medical grade honey supplies.

Overall, the objective of the supply programme is to assess and manage every stage in the production of the honey, and ensure full traceability back to the hive (_Figure 6.2_) and collection environment. The quality systems and standards developed ensure that the final product requirements for minimal levels of microbiological, chemical and physical contamination of the honey are met. We have conducted full audits on each accredited supplier against the standards at the implementation stages, and we will continue an audit monitoring programme to ensure continual compliance throughout each honey production season (*Figure 6.3*).

Systems and standards

We have set the systems and standards for production of honey, based on international criteria for raw material supply for medical device manufacturing. The systems are also designed for preventing contamination that cannot be removed afterwards, and for the prevention of natural quality deterioration/loss during storage. The honey quality aspects that need to be considered to meet the standards are contamination issues (physical, chemical and microbiological), sensory quality (smell, taste, and colour) and other quality issues such as moisture content, honey fermentation, sugar crystals and Manuka honey gelling character.

Resource management

The honey supply programme has been designed with landowners who are actively engaged with our organisation and our honey suppliers in the production of medical grade honey. The Manuka resource land management standards are based on 'organic' land use programmes and require that landowners work closely with beekeepers in all aspects of land management and honey harvesting. In return, accredited landowners who meet the specific requirements of the honey supply programme can expect to see land-usage benefits, and financial reward, from a percentage of the volume of medical grade honey produced off their land.

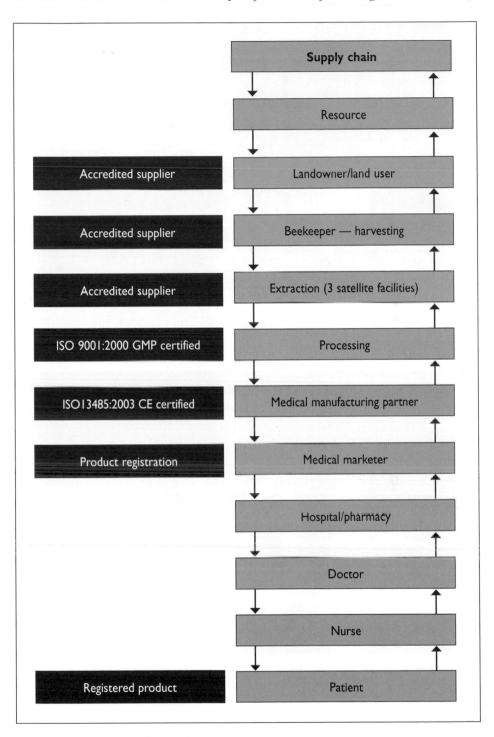

Figure 6.1: Integrated supply chain management

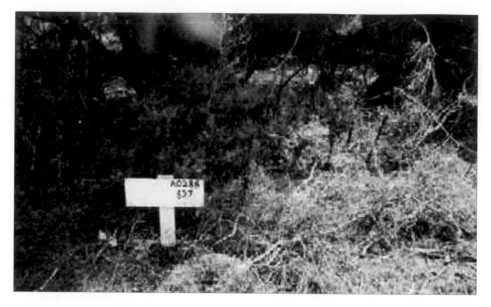

Figure 6.2: Site identification — ensuring product traceability

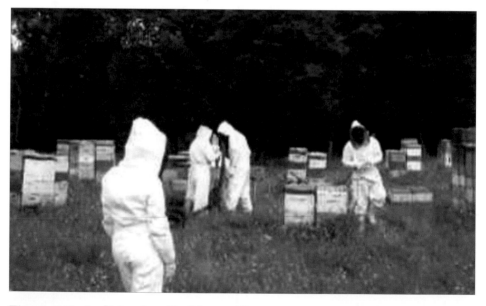

Figure 6.3: Auditing 'medical honey' harvesting — quality manager (medical)

Harvesting management

For medical grade honey harvesting, we require strict beekeeper conformance with harvest and apiary management standards. The harvest and apiary management standards involve hive site location and hive management. As part of hive management the beekeeper must use appropriate hive materials and have correct maintenance procedures. The components of the hives and their foundations must be considered, along with pest and disease management. During harvesting, smoker fuel is controlled and the bee removal process is designed in such a way that there is minimal contamination from both the equipment used and the bees themselves. Hygiene throughout the honey harvesting and transportation process is a critical factor (*Figures 6.4* and *6.5*). The harvest and apiary management standards even extend to supplemental feeding during the winter time.

Extraction standards

For medical grade honey extraction, we require extractor conformance with its extraction management standards. In summary, the standards cover critical factors of the extraction process, such as the implementation of stringent cleaning programmes to ensure hygienic extraction and the control of cross-contamination of products via appropriate extraction methods with effective wax removal procedures. Extraction facilities are required to have specifically designed and controlled air conditioning and filtration systems, along with an effective pest management programme. Processing temperatures and honey filtering systems are controlled adequately with specific requirements being placed on the filter pore size (*Figure 6.6*). Careful consideration is given to the type of drum used for raw medical grade Manuka honey, as well as the requirements of drum storage. Overall, throughout the extraction process, product traceability is still maintained to a high standard to ensure accurate trace-back if required.

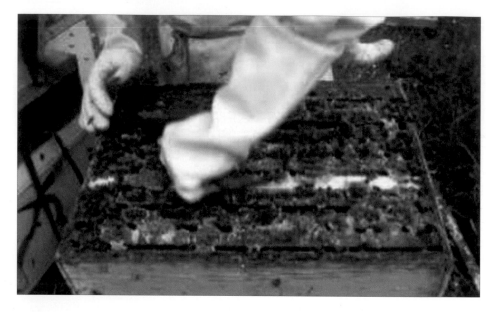

Figure 6.4: Stringent medical grade honey harvesting in practice

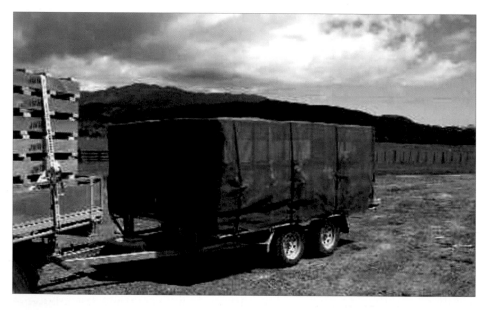

Figure 6.5: Special care for harvested honey boxes to be transported to extraction facility

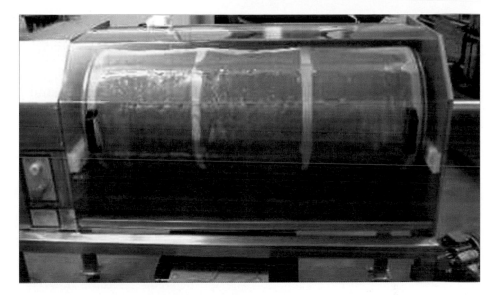

Figure 6.6: Medical grade honey filtration

Product testing regimes

We undertake strict testing regimes on the raw medical grade Manuka honey, using well developed in-house laboratory methods, as well as independent external laboratories for specific testing. The testing protocols involve rigorous analysis methods to ensure that products are safe and as pure as possible for inclusion in Medical Device manufacture.

Raw medical grade honey

The raw medical grade Manuka honey arrives from accredited suppliers in new, unused food approved drums with tamper evident seals. Each consignment is documented and recorded upon receipt with a batch number; a further number is issued individually to each drum, allowing individual traceability of the drums. Once documented and receipted into the system, the laboratory begins the sampling, testing and grading process.

The honey is sampled representatively by the in-house laboratory ready for analysis. Honey samples are then tested for the following;

moisture content, total activity, non peroxide antibacterial activity
(UMF® rating), foreign matter, sensory attributes such as Manuka typical
taste and colour, and microbiological criteria, including the total plate
count, and yeasts and moulds. Once test results are collaborated, each
drum is individually graded against the raw medical grade Manuka
honey specifications. Any drums that do not pass the raw medical grade
Manuka honey specifications are reassessed for suitability within the
therapeutic or food grade; if unsuitable for these grades the drums will
be rejected (*Table 6.1*).

Table 6.1: Examples of some of the differences between the raw medical grade honey standard compared with food and therapeutic honey grades

	Food grade	Therapeutic grade	Medical grade*
Microbiological	<100,000 cfu/g	<10,000 cfu/g	<500 cfu/g
Chemical	No chemical residues, includes plant toxins and antibiotics	No chemical residues, includes plant toxins and antibiotics	No chemical residues, includes plant toxins and antibiotics
Physical	Insoluble matter content <1.0%	Insoluble matter content <0.5%	Insoluble matter content <0.2%
Drums	New/ remanufactured with food grade linings	New with food grade linings and tamper evident	New with food grade linings and tamper evident

* Medical grade honey must be sourced from accredited suppliers who have participated and passed the accredited honey supply programme.

Processed medical grade honey

Processed medical grade honey is raw medical grade Manuka honey
formulated into a batch of product for use as an ingredient in medical
devices. We operate a quality management system which complies
with the requirements of AS/NZS ISO9001:2000 and is also Good
Manufacturing Practice certified by the New Zealand Medicines and
Medical Devices Safety Authority (MEDSAFE).

The raw honey is loaded in the factory and undergoes a minimal heat treatment process to ensure product quality. This heat treatment step has been carefully designed, implemented and validated, specific to the characteristics of honey, to ensure that the active Manuka content of the medical grade honey is unaffected.

The honey then passes through a fine filtration system and finally begins a homogenisation and pre-determined crystallisation process. Medical grade honey requires the best possible filtration techniques. We use very fine filters for the filtration of medical grade honey. Once the final stage of the process is completed the honey is pumped into new, unused drums which are fitted with a medical grade quality internal liner. This bag liner acts as the primary packaging and the honey is completely sealed within the liner to minimise or eliminate the risk of the processed medical grade honey coming into contact with the secondary packaging, the drum, and, more importantly, the external environment. At this stage the honey is tested for moisture content, pH level, heavy metal content, microbiological content, multi-pesticide residues (nil tolerance), 5-(Hydroxy methyl)-2-furfural (HMF) level, total activity and non-peroxide activity.

Once the honey has been cleared by quality personnel it is shipped to the Medical Device manufacturer where the honey is used as an ingredient for honey-impregnated Medical Devices. The Medical Device manufacturer operates a quality management system which complies with the requirements of BS EN ISO 13485 for the design and manufacture of medical products. The Medical Device Manufacturing Company also complies with the European Directives for medical devices in order to affix 'Certification European' (CE) marking on its products. Both our company and the accredited honey supply programme have been audited by the Medical Device Manufacturing Company, providing a double guarantee that the honey received as a Medical Device ingredient meets the Medical Device system requirements and specifications.

Achievements of the programme

The required quality level demanded of medical grade honey does not come without cost implications. It is this high level of quality (achieved through specific standards and systems defined by Comvita) that sets medical grade honey above all other grades of honey, and warrants the exclusive use in premium medical applications for the medical market.

Until the year 2002, it was difficult to find honey that met the stringent international Medical Device manufacturing requirements. Through workshops, education programmes, assessment and auditing processes, the accredited honey supply programme was able to produce sufficient medical grade honey in 2003 to see the first honey-impregnated Medical Devices launched onto the medical market. With the ongoing support and supply of the honey suppliers within the accredited honey supply programme, we are able to sustain the supply of raw medical grade honey, as well as to begin to extend the range of honey-impregnated Medical Devices.

References

Cooper RA, Molan PC (1999) The use of honey as an antiseptic in managing *Pseudomonas* infection. *J Wound Care* **8**: 161–4

Cooper RA, Molan PC, Harding KG (1999) Antibacterial activity of honey against strains of *Staphylococcus aureus* from infected wounds. *J R Soc Med* **92**: 283–5

Cooper RA, Molan PC, Krishnamoorthy L, Harding KG (2001) Manuka honey used to heal a recalcitrant surgical wound. *Eur J Clin Microbiol Infect Dis* **20**: 758–9

Molan PC (1998) A brief review of honey as a clinical dressing. *Primary Intention* **6**: 148–58

Molan PC (2001) Honey for the treatment of wounds and burns. *New Ethical J* July: 1–16

Molan PC, Allen KL (1996) The effect of gamma-irradiation on the antibacterial activity of honey. *J Pharm Pharmacol* **48**: 1206–09

Mossel DAA (1980) Honey for necrotic breast ulcers. *Lancet* **ii**: 1091

Snowdon JA, Cliver DO (1996) Microorganisms in honey. *Int J Microbiol* **31**: 1–26

Snowdon JA (1999) The microbiology of honey — meeting your buyers' specifications (Why they do what they do). *Am Bee J* **xx**: 51–9

Chapter 7

The use of Leptospermum honey on chronic wounds in breast care

Val Robson, Lee Martin and Rose Cooper

The following case studies illustrate how honey-based wound dressings were successfully incorporated into the care plan of two patients with breast lesions. In the first case, wound breakdown followed breast reduction surgery and, in the second, necrosis developed after radiotherapy. In both cases the wounds were refractory to 'first line' treatment but resolved with honey. Whilst there is a large body of evidence to support the use of honey in other wound types, there are few reports in breast care (Mossel, 1980; Keast-Butler, 1980).

Case study 1: control of malodour in a breast wound

Miss A was twenty-two years old when she was referred to a breast surgeon in April 2003 with pain and asymmetry due to benign changes in her left breast. At review, six weeks later, following a normal ultrasound scan and treatment with danazol, Miss A was resolute in her wish for breast reduction and was listed for surgery, that was performed in February 2004. Her breast was reduced using a superior medial pedicle technique removing 236 gms of normal breast tissue, with minimal skin tension on the wounds. Miss A made an uneventful recovery and was discharged the following day. At two weeks the wounds appeared to be healing well and at the six-week review, the T-junction had healed without problem. However, there had been some breakdown of the wound at the nipple/

vertical incision junction, even though healthy granulation tissue was present within the wound. Two weeks later the wound had deteriorated further. At initial referral to the wound clinic, although satisfied with improved breast symmetry, the unhealed wound was severely impacting on Miss A's lifestyle. She refused to look at the wound or apply dressings and she found the wound exudate distressing. She felt that the wound was malodorous and was convinced that other people were aware of the odour. Unable to accept these problems, Miss A would tolerate only dry dressings and left the wound care entirely to her mother. At this time, the wound contained some granulation tissue with small areas of necrosis and slough (*Figure 7.1*).

The initial goal at the outset of treatment was to control the odour as Miss A found this the most distressing symptom of the wound.

The patient was advised to shower daily and then apply Medihoney™ (Medihoney Pty Ltd) at a depth of 3mm with an adhesive foam dressing to protect and secure. Two weeks later (*Figure 7.2*), the necrosis and slough had been cleared from the wound and was replaced with healthy granulation tissue. Miss A still refused to look at the wound but agreed that the malodour had completely resolved. At one month (*Figure 7.3*) the wound contained healthy granulation tissue and Miss A was able to deal with the dressing regime herself. The wound continued to improve and, at review, sixteen weeks after recruitment to the trial, she reported that the wound had healed three weeks previously.

Miss A had found honey an acceptable dressing, and was particularly pleased that she was able to shower daily during treatment. She reported that the odour control resulting from the use of honey in the dressing regime was of paramount importance to her.

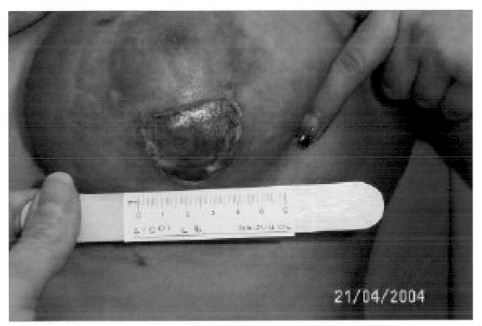

Figure 7.1: Breast wound at the start of treatment with honey. Note the presence of slough and necrotic tissue

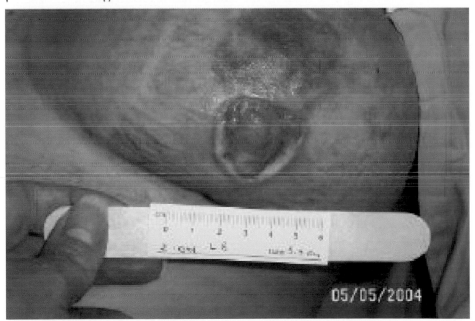

Figure 7.2: Two weeks after commencement of treatment. The wound is showing signs of healing, the necrosis has resolved and the wound margins have progressed

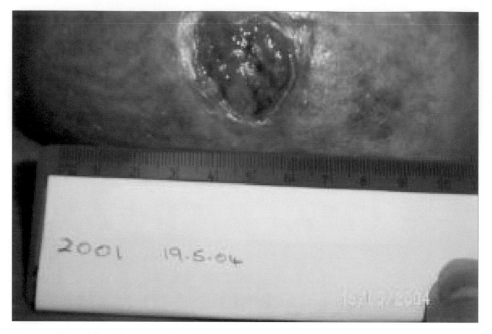

Figure 7.3: After four weeks of treatment with honey, the wound is showing positive signs of healing, the slough has resolved and re-epithelialisation is well underway

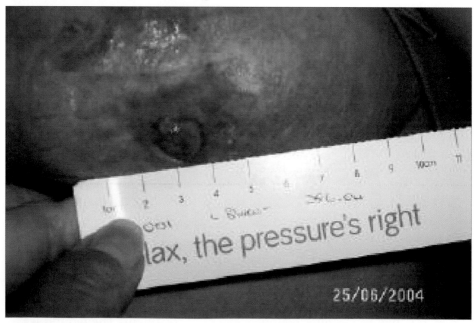

Figure 7.4: After nine weeks of treatment with honey, the wound has reduced in size

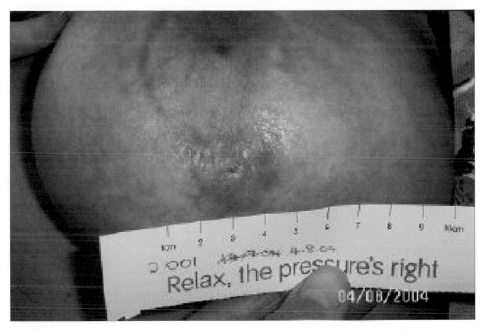

Figure 7.5: The wound at healing (fifteen weeks after the start of treatment with honey)

Casc study 2: management of radio necrosis

Mrs B was an eighty-year-old widowed, self-caring lady who enjoyed an active social life. In 1970 she was diagnosed with carcinoma of her left breast and underwent a Patey mastectomy, followed by a course of radiation therapy. In February 2001 she was referred by her GP for surgical consultation with a hyperkeratotic lesion of the upper sternal region that had been present for two years. A biopsy confirmed a viral wart and chronic radiation dermatitis. On return to clinic two weeks later, there was slough present in the wound and she was prescribed Augmentin®. The area healed after thirteen months, only to re-ulcerate a few months later, when she was referred to a plastic surgeon. Dressings were prescribed and the patient was referred to community nurses for car e.

In September 2003, Mrs B was referred to the breast clinic because the ulcerated area had enlarged. It was approximately 4 cm x 3 cm with necrotic bone and costal cartilage observable at the base of the wound The wound was dressed with 1% silver sulfadiazine cream and a course of ciprofloxacin prescribed. Mrs B was also reviewed at this time by the oncologist. A full computed tomography (CT) scan revealed an ulcer on either side of the sternum with bony destruction. There was no focal mass lesion. The appearances were in keeping with either radiation necrosis or direct neoplastic invasion, but a biopsy confirmed radiation necrosis. The underlying dermis showed areas of necrosis, together with granulation tissue formation and dense mixed acute and chronic inflammatory cell infiltration, including numerous plasma cells. There was no evidence of malignancy.

Delayed radiotherapy ulcers are more common than acute ulcers and tend to be the result of ischaemia from changes in small arteries and arterioles; they heal slowly and may persist for many years (Mendelsohn *et al*, 2002). Late skin effects due to radiation therapy occur months to years after irradiation and are manifested by scaling, atrophy, telangiectasia, subcutaneous fibrosis, and necrosis. These symptoms may evolve and increase in severity for many years (Heggie *et al*, 2002), depending upon numerous factors. In general, high radiation doses (both daily and total) induce severe reactions in patients. Treatment field size is also an influence: the larger the area being irradiated, the less tolerance the skin has due to an increase in the area of capillary obstruction. Occlusion of the arteriocapillary circulation results in tissue infarction, leading to sclerosis and eventually fibrosis. This blocks the transport of vital nutrients to the tissues. Skin reactions are particularly evident in skin folds and areas subjected to pressure, such as bony prominences (Korinko and Yurick, 1997).

In January 2004, Mrs B was referred to the wound clinic. The wound was exuding thick offensive pus and necrotic bone and cartilage was visible within the wound. A wound swab confirmed mixed growth including *Staphylococcus aureus* and *Bacteroides spp*. This latter organism is an anaerobe known to contribute to wound malodour (Bowler *et al*, 1999). The patient was feeling well, although depressed and rarely left her home. The wound was being packed daily with an alginate rope and Mrs B was concerned that the area would never heal (*Figure 7.6*).

There were several problems to address following assessment. Mrs B was clearly finding it difficult to cope with a wound having such profound affect upon her life. The position of the wound meant that she was constantly aware of its odour. It was painful and the exudate leaked through the dressing regularly. The peri-wound area was sore and excoriated.

Mrs B was referred to the district nurses to increase the frequency of dressings to daily. The dressing regime was to apply skin protection

(Cavilon™, 3M Ltd) to the surrounding area and to pack the wound with an alginate rope (Algisite™, Smith and Nephew) soaked in Medihoney™ (Medihoney Pty Ltd) secured with a foam adhesive dressing. Progress was monitored at regular intervals (*Figures 7.7–7.10*) at the wound clinic.

After twenty-seven weeks of treatment (*Figure 7.10*), the wound had improved but complete healing was not achieved. A wound swab at this stage confirmed the presence of *Proteus* species and anaerobic cocci.

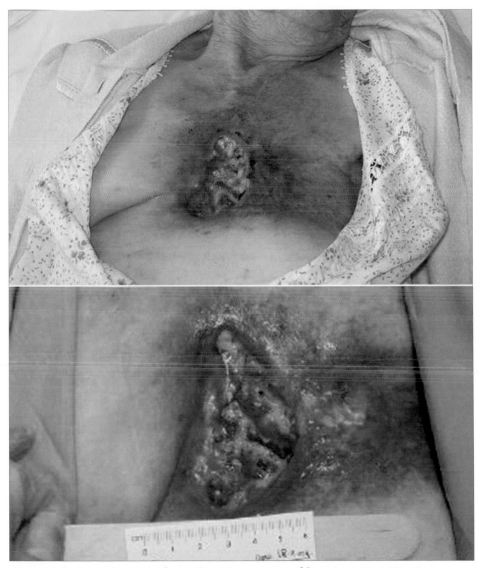

Figure 7.6: Mrs B's wound at commencement of honey treatment

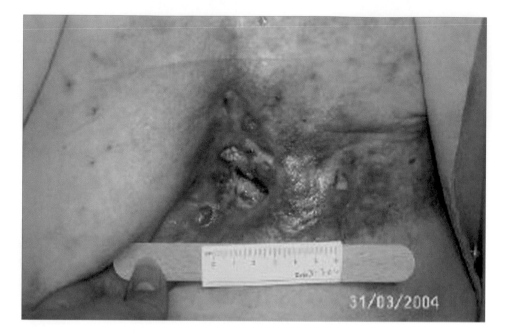

Figure 7.7: The wound after six weeks of treatment

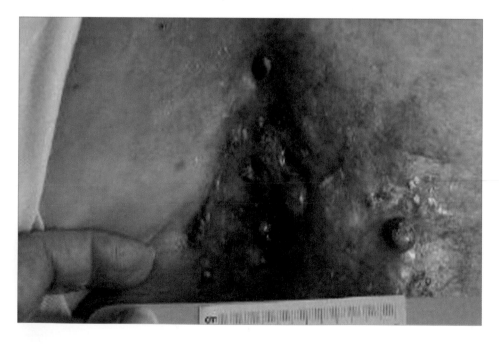

Figure 7.8: The wound after twelve weeks of treatment

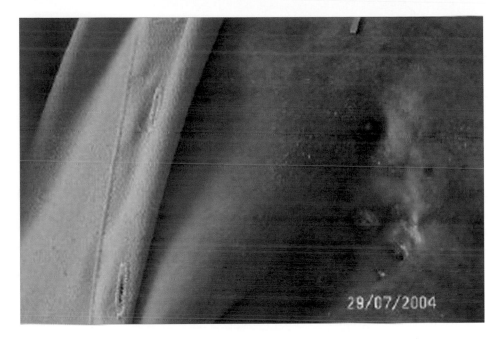

Figure 7.9: The wound after twenty-three weeks of treatment

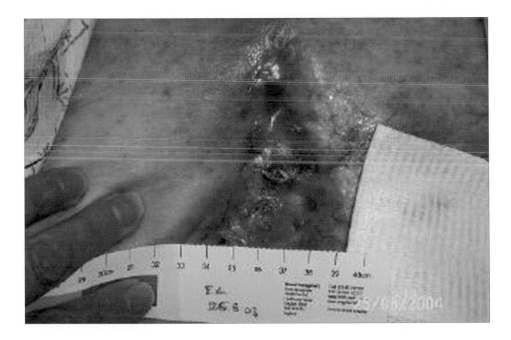

Figure 7.10: Twenty-seven weeks from commencement of treatment

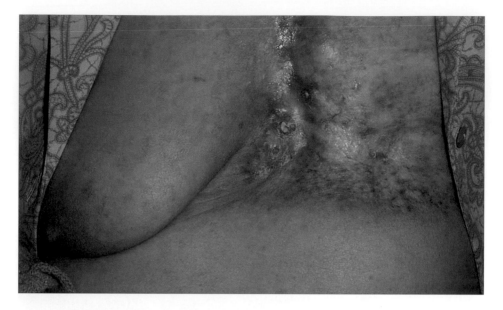

Figure 7.11: Photograph of healed wound

Discussion

Initially, the patients in the studies were pessimistic about wound treatment with honey but were willing to accept, what some may consider, an unconventional therapy. Both patients found the use of honey acceptable, which is consistent with previous reports of patient satisfaction with honey dressings (Dunford and Hanano, 2004; Robson, 2003; Cooper *et al*, 2001). Although initial problems with leakage from dressings were experienced, as the honey reached body temperature and became more fluid, the problem was easily resolved when a satisfactory secondary dressing was used. The availability of newer dressings impregnated with honey, with the capacity to hold wound exudate, will pre-empt this situation in the future.

Dressings were initially changed daily for both patients and the frequency between changes was extended for Miss A as healing proceeded. In comparison to conventional dressings which are designed to remain in-situ for several days, this treatment may seem uneconomical, but the ease of application of honey allows some patients to manage their own dressing changes, thereby reducing district nursing time. As Mrs B was already receiving daily dressings from the district nursing team prior to the application of honey dressings, this did not represent any increased costs. Molan (1999) has stated that the frequency of dressing changes must depend on the extent of dilution of honey by exudation, which normally reduces with time. Loss of fluid from a wound will reduce oedema and pain, and may account for some of the anti-inflammatory properties attributed to honey.

Mrs B had complained of pain within the wound before the start of honey treatment but found it to be diminished when honey was used. There are reports of patients who complain of pain on the initial application of honey and some have experienced continuous pain (Dunford and Hanano, 2004).

Neither of the patients in these case studies reported pain during treatment with honey.

Wound malodour can have serious effects on patient morale and the control of wound odour was critical for both patients reported in these case studies. Early eradication of this problem, as well as reduction in the size of the wound, had positive effects on both patients. There are many reports of honey having a rapid effect on the presence of malodour within a wound (Dunford and Hanano, 2004; Cooper _et al_, 2002a, b; Efem, 1988; Alcaraz and Kelly, 2002; Kingsley, 2001 are a few of the many such reports).

Honey has been found to inhibit major wound pathogens (Cooper _et al_, 2002a, b; Molan, 1999; Willix _et al_, 1992; Cooper and Molan, 1999), even when diluted by high levels of exudate in a wound. The eradication of bacteria from Mrs B's wound was not achieved on this occasion.

The psychological and emotional burden of a chronic wound is always debilitating; it affects patients' self-esteem, as well as having adverse effects on their daily lives. Effects often extend to employers and to other family members. Holistic patient assessment, together with the correct dressing selection to manage and improve the condition of a wound is vital. The healthcare professional, too, may become frustrated when well-proven and researched conventional therapies fail to have a beneficial impact on the wound.

In these two cases, 'appropriate' modern wound treatments had failed to promote healing, but both the patients experienced complete healing with honey.

Acknowledgements

The honey used in all the case studies is MediHoney™ presented in 30g tubes that had been gamma irradiated without affecting the antibacterial activity. MediHoney™ is produced in Australia by Medihoney Pty Ltd and is a standardised mix of antibacterial honeys including Australian and New Zealand *Leptospermum spp*.

Data for all these case studies is collected using the Leg Ulcer Telemedicine Medicine System (LUTMS), designed by Good Hope Hospital, West Midlands. LUTMS is a dedicated, secure, shared electronic patient record. The LUTMS has been designed to allow the incorporation of colour digital images in the electronic patient record. The LUTMS includes ulcer size measurement and automatically plots ulcer-healing rate. Information regarding the LUTMS can be obtained by contacting simon.dodds@goodhope.nhs.uk.

Study support

MediHoney Pty Ltd, Australia
University Hospital Aintree
University Hospital Aintree Research Committee
The Florence Nightingale Foundation
The Florence Nightingale Council
The Huntleigh Foundation

References

Alcaraz A, Kelly J (2002) Treatment of an infected venous ulcer with honey dressings. *Br J Nurs* **11**:13: 859–66

Bowler PG, Davies BJ, Jones SA (1999) Microbial involvement in chronic wound malodour. *J Wound Care* **8**(5): 216–18

Cooper R, Molan PC (1999) The use of honey as an antiseptic in managing *Pseudomonas* infection. *J Wound Care* **8**(4): 161–4

Cooper RA, Molan PC, Krishnamoorthy L, Harding KG (2001) Manuka honey used to heal a recalcitrant surgical wound. *Eur J Infect Dis* **20**: 758–9

Cooper RA, Halas E, Molan PC (2002a) The efficacy of honey in inhibiting strains of *Pseudomonas aeruginosa* from infected burns. *J Burn Care Rehab* **23**(6): 366–70

Cooper RA, Molan PC, Harding KG (2002b) The sensitivity of honey of Gram-positive cocci of clinical significance isolated from wounds. *J Appl Microbiol* **93**(5): 857–63

Dunford C, Hanano R (2004) Acceptability to patients of a honey dressing for non-healing venous leg ulcers. *J Wound Care* **13**(5): 193–7

Efem SE (1988) Clinical observations on the wound healing properties of honey. *Br J Surg* **75**: 679–81

Heggie S, Bryant GP, Tripcony L (2002) A phase III study of the efficacy of topical aloe vera gel on irradiated breast tissue. *Cancer Nurs* **25**(6): 442–51

Keast-Butler J (1980) Honey for malignant breast ulcers. *Lancet* **2**(8198): 809

Kingsley A(2001) The use of honey in the treatment of infected wounds: case studies. *Br J Nurs* **10**(22): 13–20

Korinko A, Yurick A (1997) Maintaining skin integrity during radiation therapy. *Am J Nurs* **97**(2): 40–4

Mendelsohn FA, Divino CM, Reis ED, Kerstein MD (2002) Wound care after radiation therapy. *Adv Skin Wound Care* **15**(5): 216–24

Molan PC, Allen KL (1996) The effect of gamma-irradiation on the antibacterial activity of honey. *J Pharmacol* **48**: 1206–09

Molan PC (1999) The role of honey in the management of wounds. *J Wound Care* **8**(8): 415–8

Mossel DA (1980) Honey for necrotic breast ulcers. *Lancet* **2**(8203) 1091

Robson V (2003) Leptospermum honey used as a debriding agent. *Nurse* **2**(11): 66–8

Willix D, Molan PC, Harfoot C (1992) A comparison of the sensitivity of wound infecting species of bacteria to the antibacterial activity of Manuka honey and other honey. *J Appl Bacteriol* **73**: 388–94

CHAPTER 8

THE USE OF HONEY IN WOUND MANAGEMENT

Cheryl Dunford

Part I: The use of honey in the treatment of meningococcal skin lesions

A preliminary report of this case study was first published in April 2000 in the *Nursing Times* (Dunford, 2000). It had a huge impact and was immediately picked up by the media. The fact that such a natural agent as honey could be responsible for healing such devastating lesions in a young adult so badly affected by meningococcal septicaemia made it newsworthy. There followed numerous national and local newspaper reports as well as TV and radio appearances both nationally and also in New Zealand and Australia. This positive attention no doubt also helped the patient, referred to as Jem, come to terms with his experience. It also introduced honey as a healing agent to the general public and health practitioners alike, and began the significant public and professional interest in honey that has grown in recent years.

Patient history

Jem was fifteen when he contracted meningococcal septicaemia. His was a classic presentation of feeling unwell with myalgia and nausea for a few hours before collapsing. Meningoccocal disease is caused by the bacterium *Neisseria meningitidis* that is found in human nasopharyngeal tract. Under certain conditions, such as concomitant viral infection or reduced immune response, penetration of the mucosa leading to outgrowth in the bloodstream can occur. Further information on this condition is provided in *Figure 8.1*.

❖ Bacteraemia manifests first as acute fever, low back pain, generalised aches, and without shock.

❖ Fulminant meningococcal sepsis (FMS) with shock and disseminated intravascular coagulation may develop without signs of meningitis.

❖ The mortality rate from FMS is 20–80%.

❖ Skin haemorrhages are characteristic of meningococcal disease.

❖ Skin and limb necrosis requiring amputation or plastic surgery is seen in 10–20% of patients.

❖ Meningococcal disease does not consist only of meningitis!

Figure 8.1: Features of meningococcal septicaemia (van Deuren *et al*, 2000)

Jem required immediate resuscitation on admission to hospital and was given full system support and ventilation in intensive care for the next thirty days. Jem developed fulminant meningococcal septicaemia (FMS) as a result of the massive outgrowth of toxins. This resulted in both adult respiratory distress syndrome and acute renal failure. Extensive haemorrhagic skin lesions (ecchymoses) appeared on his lower limbs and peripheral necrosis of both his hands and feet developed. Despite attempts at salvage, bilateral transtibial amputation together with amputation of distal and middle phalanges of both hands was necessary. Multiple skin grafts were harvested and applied to the residual limbs. After two months of treatment Jem was transferred to a regional burns and plastics unit. By this time he had developed a Grade 3 pressure ulcer on his left buttock and he was nutritionally compromised.

The amputation sites on Jem's hands healed without incident but there was to follow six months of skin grafting to his legs, which in most cases proved unsuccessful. This resulted in a number of non-healing donor sites. Pain was a major issue in Jem's care. Despite the administration of Oramorph®, dihydrocodeine and diazepam for dressing changes, pain was never properly controlled, therefore, the majority of dressing changes (approximately twice weekly) were undertaken under general anaesthetic. A high-protein, high-calorie diet was started which was supplemented by overnight gastric feeding.

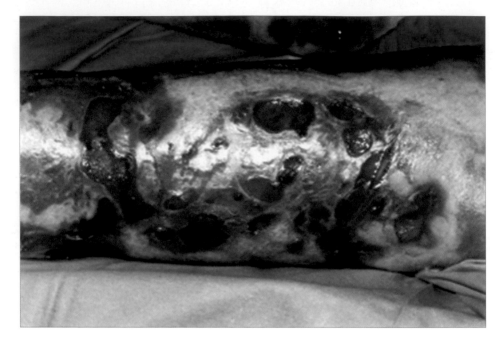

Figure 8.2: Infected meningococcal lesion prior to honey dressings

The skin lesions were initially dressed using paraffin Tulle dressings (Jelonet™, Smith and Nephew) with alginate dressings (Kaltostat™, ConvaTec) to the donor sites. A hydrocolloid dressing (Granuflex™, ConvaTec) was applied to the pressure ulcer. Swabs from his lower legs showed heavy growth of *Pseudomonas spp*, *Staphylococcus aureus* and *Enterococcus spp*. Topical silver sulfadiazine 1% cream was applied as a consequence, but proved ineffective in eliminating the bioburden present in the lesions. Even after copious amounts of analgesia and soaking in a bath, the dressings were still difficult to remove. This meant that dressing and wound debris began to accumulate increasing the risk of infection. All lesions remained static.

It was at this stage that a referral to the tissue viability team was made. Following assessment it was decided to introduce a multi-layer dressing (Tenderwet™, Paul Hartmann AG) with the aim of providing atraumatic dressing removal together with effective wound cleansing. Despite initial favourable results, the frequency of dressing change required for this product proved impracticable.

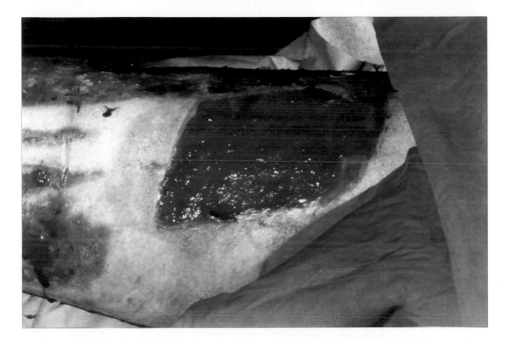

Figure 8.3: A failed donor site prior to treatment

At this point a new approach was necessary. Gamma irradiated absorbent dressing pads impregnated with 25–35g of active Manuka honey (UMF 13) were obtained and initially applied to Jem's right leg only. The left leg continued to be dressed as before as a form of control. Again, a general anaesthetic was used to dress the lesions at three-day intervals. Wound swabs were taken at the start of the honey dressings and at regular intervals throughout the treatment period. The rationale for the use of honey dressings is shown in Table 8.1.

Within a few days the right leg showed signs of epithelialisation with a corresponding reduction in wound bacteria. Following this, all lesions were dressed using honey, including the pressure ulcer. The _Pseudomonas spp_ and _Enterococcus spp_ were both eliminated within a few weeks of honey dressings. Interestingly enough, _Staphylococcus aureus_ remained throughout the healing process without appearing to hinder it. It was also noticed that all traces of odour from the lesions were eliminated within the first dressing change. However, it was not fully appreciated by anyone at this stage how much of an impact the odour and its associations were having on Jem. The rate of healing and reduction in odour allowed Jem to gain more control over his situation and within a few weeks he was able to undertake dressing changes using a mixture of Entonox® and oxygen. The honey dressings did not adhere and were easily removed with use of a shower trolley. The epithelialisation continued and further skin grafts were applied six weeks after starting the honey treatment that this time proved successful after many previous failed attempts.

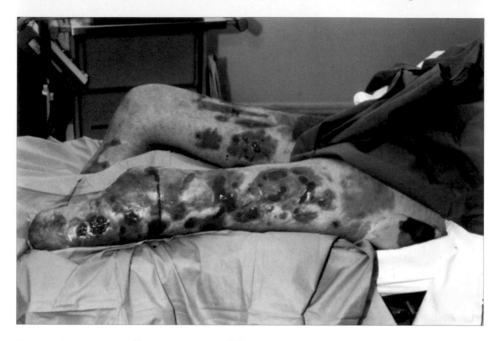

Figure 8.4: Signs of improvement following one week of honey dressings

Within ten weeks all lesions, including the pressure ulcer, were completely healed and Jem was able to be discharged and to begin his very successful rehabilitation programme. Not only did the lesions finally heal within a relatively short period of time, but also the resultant scar tissue was of good quality with no evidence of hypertrophic scarring. As with burn injuries, contracture and hypertrophic scarring can be a long-term problem in meningococcal lesions.

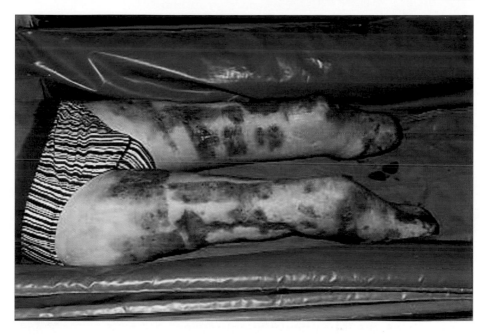

Figure 8.5: Decrease in bacterial loading evident following four weeks of treatment

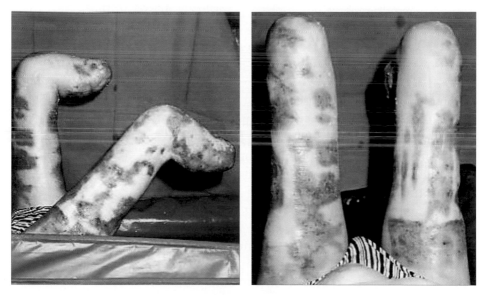

Figure 8.6 a and b: Signs of significant improvement with epithelialisation present at week six

Discussion

Jem's was the first reported case of using honey for infected skin lesions on multiple meningococcal lesions. An excellent clinical outcome was achieved, highlighting the effectiveness of honey in the various stages of wound healing as described in *Table 8.1*. The honey was able to eliminate the *Pseudomonas spp* that had proved so problematic for many months. An additional outcome from using honey dressings was the thorough wound bed preparation that facilitated successful skin grafting after many failures. Although the antimicrobial and anti-inflammatory properties of honey did play a significant part in 'kick starting' the healing process, they were probably not the factors that helped to turn the whole situation around for Jem. Prior to the application of honey, dressing changes had been a time of major anxiety and distress for Jem. What we had failed to realise was the impact that the smell of his wounds was having on him, as the smell was not considered particularly malodorous by those involved in his care. The original case study included an account by Jem in which he states the following, 'one of the first things I noticed [after using the honey dressing] was the smell wasn't nearly so bad. I'm not saying that it was worse than the pain, because the pain was bad, but the smell was one of the things that bothered me most'. Jem had had the traumatic experience of having to live with his decaying limbs and their smell before the decision was made to amputate them. The association between smell and emotion is well recognised. The smell of hospitals can cause major anxiety in some people and the smell of cabbage, associated with school dinners, can spoil the enjoyment of a meal. By eliminating the smell, Jem did not have such a strong trigger for his anxiety and was able to gain further control of his situation. This also allowed him to gain better control of his own pain relief. For many patients, particularly with non-healing wounds, the elimination of odour is of major importance. The ability of honey to do this effectively and quickly should not be underestimated.

There may be a place for using honey earlier on in the treatment of meningococcal lesions. Oedema increases the risk of purpuric skin lesions deteriorating into necrotic areas. The ability of honey to reduce inflammation and oedema could prove advantageous at this stage, and as demonstrated so well in this case, could reduce any associated malodour.

Table 8.1: Rationale for use of honey dressings

Clinical action	Mode of action
Odour elimination	Glucose metabolism by the infecting bacteria to lactic acid instead of amino acids from serum and dead cells resulting in ammonia and sulphur compounds
Antimicrobial activity	❖ Production of hydrogen peroxide, action of non-peroxide components (phyto-chemicals) and acidity ❖ Stimulation of immune response including ß-lymphocytes, neutrophils and cytokines. Supply of glucose for respiratory burst and for energy production in macrophages
Anti-inflammatory activity	❖ Decrease in leukocytes ❖ Inhibition of reactive oxygen species (ROI) production as a result of antioxidant activity ❖ Suppression of inflammatory process through scavenging of free radicals by antioxidants
Reduction in pain	❖ Anti-inflammatory properties, as above ❖ Moist wound healing environment ❖ Non-adherence, resulting in atraumatic removal
Stimulation of healing	❖ Increased phagocytosis due to stimulatory effect of honey on macrophages ❖ Increased autolytic debridement due to osmolarity effects ❖ Increased angiogenesis, collagen synthesis, granulation and epithelialisation as a result of honey components and low hydrogen peroxide production with antioxidant protection that modifies proteins important to cell growth
Reduction in scarring	Suppression of inflammatory process, as above

Reference: American National Honey Board, 2003

References

American National Honey Board (2003) *Honey — Health and Therapeutic Qualities*. American National Honey Board, USA

Dunford C, Cooper R, Molan P (2000) Using honey as a dressing for infected skin lesions. *Nursing Times Plus* **96**(14): 7–9

van Deuren M, Brandtzaeg P, van der Meer J (2000) Update on meningococcal disease with emphasis on pathophysiology and clinical management. *J Clin Microbiological Rev* **13**(1): 144–66

Part II: The use of honey in venous leg ulcers

This section illustrates the effectiveness of honey by use of a single case study examining an unusual leg ulceration presentation.

A summary of the reported wound healing properties of honey is shown in *Table 8.2*. The most important of these being its antimicrobial properties.

Table 8.2: Reported wound healing properties of honey		
Property	**Anticipated clinical**	**Mode of action**
Antimicrobial activity	❖ Inhibits wide range of Gram negative and Gram positive bacteria and fungi ❖ Deodorises wounds ❖ Prevention of cross-contamination through protective barrier	❖ Production of hydrogen peroxide and action of phytochemicals ❖ Stimulation of immune system ❖ Glucose metabolism by bacteria to produce non-odorous lactic acid (instead of malodorous ammonia and sulphur compounds) ❖ High viscosity creates physical barrier
Anti-inflammatory activity	❖ Reduction in oedema ❖ Reduction in pain ❖ Reduction in scarring	❖ High osmolarity leading to fluid outflow and creation of moist healing environment ❖ Decrease in leukocytes associated with inflammation ❖ Inhibition of reactive oxygen intermediates (ROI) production as a result of antioxidant production
Stimulation of wound healing	❖ Increased autolytic debridement and phagocytosis ❖ Increased angiogenesis and formation of granulation tissue ❖ Cell proliferation ❖ Collagen synthesis ❖ Re-epithelialisation	❖ Stimulatory effect of honey proteins on macrophages ❖ Increased debriding by moist environment and outflow of lymph and nutrients ❖ Increased oxygen supply secondary to the outflow of lymph and acidity of honey ❖ Controlled low hydrogen peroxide production stimulates cell production

Adapted from American National Honey Board, 2003

Case study

The patient was an eighty-five-year-old lady who presented with a twenty-month history of venous leg ulceration, presenting as numerous small ulcers present on her right leg. The largest of these ulcers measured 1.8 cm in length and 1.1 cm in breadth (*Figure 8.7*). She was otherwise fit and healthy with no physical problems of note. Her only medication being paracetamol for general aches and pains. Her ankle/brachial pressure index was 0.98 in each leg and she was treated using a three-layer compression system in conjunction with a simple non-adherent dressing. Investigations, including full blood count, liver function, thyroid function and calcium and parathyroid hormone levels were all within normal range. Community nursing staff at a local leg ulcer clinic, which she attended on a weekly basis, managed her leg ulceration.

The patient also presented with subcutaneous calcium deposits that appeared as small, hard lumps palpable beneath the skin of both lower legs. The calcium deposits also presented within the ulcer beds where they appeared as hard, irregular shaped lumps, which were attached to the wound bed (*Figure 8.7*). There was evidence of chronic inflammation in each of the ulcers, possibly as a consequence of the foreign body reaction to the deposits. The wound margins were poorly defined and the ulcer beds were also superficially sloughy. She experienced mild to discomforting pain as a result of the ulcers, which was effectively controlled with paracetamol. There had been no evidence of any reduction in size of the ulcers during her visits to the leg ulcer clinic.

Subcutaneous calcification or calcinosis cutis is the abnormal deposition of calcium and phosphate in the skin (Chave *et al*, 2001). The presence of these calcium deposits in soft tissues may lead to non-healing chronic ulcers (Brietstein *et al*, 2002). There are a number of causes for this condition, which have been categorised into dystrophic, metatastic, idiopathic or iatrogenic (Walsh and Fairley, 1995). Metastatic calciphylaxis involves abnormalities of calcium and/or phosphate metabolism, which leads to microvascular calcification and is a serious but rare complication of end-stage renal disease (Burkhart *et al*, 1999). Dystrophic calcinosis cutis can be seen in patients with venous hypertension and venous ulceration where it is confined to the soft tissues and does not involve the vessels. Chave *et al* (2001) suggest that calcification in this instance may be a result of the inflammation from venous leakage. This condition is rarely reported in the literature. Treatment measures are confined to surgical excision on the deposits and treatment of the underlying venous hypertension.

Prior to commencement of honey dressings, the patient had had to attend a vascular clinic every three months to have the deposits removed from the ulcer beds using sharp debridement. Unless removed on a regular basis, the deposits tended to merge together and so increase in size. The debridement process often resulted in pain and bleeding and the patient disliked the experience.

The patient was recruited into a small clinical trial designed to determine the acceptability of honey for non-healing leg ulcers (Dunford and Hanano, 2004). Honey dressings were applied on a weekly basis under the existing compression system. Assessment was undertaken every two weeks for a total of twelve weeks, in which perceived levels of pain, odour and patient satisfaction with the dressings were monitored.

It was noted on the first assessment that pieces of calcium were evident on the honey-dressing pad on removal. This finding was not anticipated. This atraumatic removal of deposits continued with further use of honey dressings. In addition, the condition of the ulcer beds improved with a reduction in size, local surrounding inflammation and slough. There was no reported increase in pain as a result of using the honey dressings and the ulcers remained odour free. Patient satisfaction with the dressings was understandably high, as the traumatic experience of surgical debridement of the deposits was no longer required.

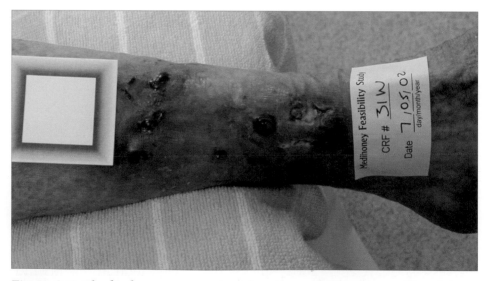

Figure 8.7: The limb on presentation showing multiple ulcers with calcium deposits

❖ Only use wound care honey which has been sterilised using gamma irradiation.

❖ Use sufficient honey for the wound in question. More may be required if the wound is large, heavily exudating or is sloughy or necrotic.

❖ Expect wound exudate to increase initially, so prepare patient for this and ensure that resources are available for dressing changes.

❖ Choose a honey preparation that is suitable for the wound, eg. gel or impregnated dressing.

❖ If wound is heavily exudating use a suitable secondary dressing to prevent maceration of surrounding skin.

❖ If packing a wound choose an appropriate dressing (eg. mannuronic acid alginate) to use in conjunction with the honey.

❖ Honey can cause a transient stinging and drawing sensation — make patients aware and ensure effective pain control prior to application.

❖ Honey staining can occur to skin but this is easily removed using soap and water.

Figure 8.8: Factors to consider when using honey dressings

Discussion

Not all patients with leg ulcers respond to recognised treatment regimes (eg. compression therapy). Unfortunately, for some leg ulcer patients the end point objective of total wound healing is not always achieved. This is a patient group where quality of life issues, such as pain and odour, are well documented (Douglas, 2001). This case study has focused on one such patient where total wound healing was an unrealistic outcome. The use of honey, not only resulted in a reduction in local inflammation and improved wound bed, but also the atraumatic removal of calcified deposits. This was an unexpected but very positive outcome. It is felt that the osmotic potential and viscosity of the honey helped to remove the deposits. This may account for the ability of honey to debride sloughy tissue and to assist in the removal of dirt.

Clinical observations suggest honey holds significant promise as an effective treatment in the management of wounds and that this is an area worthy of further research.

The case study presented in Part II of this chapter, is reproduced by kind permission of *Professional Nurse* **20**(8).

References

Brietstein R, Sonkin D, Hubbard C (2002) Non-hyperparathyroid wound calcifications: Two case presentations and literature review. *Wounds* **14**(4): 136–41

Burkhart C, Burkhart C, Mian A (1999) Calciphylaxis: A case report and review of literature. *Wounds* **11**(2): 58–61

Cavanagh D, Beazely J, Ostapowicz F (1970) Radical operation for carcinoma of the vulva. A new approach to wound healing. *J Obstet Gynaecol Br Commonwealth* **77**(11): 103–40

Chave T, Varma S, Knight A (2001) Dystrophic calcinosis cutis in venous ulcers: a cause of treatment failure. *Br J Dermatol* **145**: 349–73

Cooper R, Molan P, Harding K (2002) The sensitivity of honey of Gram-positive cocci of clinical significance isolated from wounds. *J Appl Microbiol* **93**: 857–63

Cooper R, Molan P, Harding K (1999) Antibacterial activity of honey against strains of *Staphylococcus aureus* isolated form infected wounds. *J R Soc Med* **92**: 283–5

Douglas V (2001) Living with a chronic leg ulcer: an insight into patients' experiences and feelings. *J Wound Care* **10**: 355–60

Dunford C, Hanano R (2004) Patient acceptability and tolerance of Medihoney™ in the management of non-healing leg ulcers. *J Wound Care* **13**(5): 193–7

Efem, S (1993) Recent advances in the management of Fournier's gangrene: preliminary observations. *Surgery* **113**(2): 200–4

Heibling A, Peter C, Berchtold E, Bogdanov S, Muller U (1992) Allergy to honey: relation to pollen and honey bee allergy. *Allergy* **47**(1):41–9

Jones R (2002) Honey and healing through the ages. In: Munn P, ed. *Honey and Healing.* IBRA, Cardiff, UK: 1–4

Lord A (2000) Sweet healing. *The New Scientist* **168**(2259): 32–6

Molan P (1999) The role of honey in the management of wounds. *J Wound Care* **8**(8): 415–8

Molan P (2001) Why honey is effective as a medicine 2. The scientific explanation of its effects. In: Munn P, ed. *Honey and Healing*. IBRA, Cardiff, UK: 14–26

Molan P, Betts J (2004) Clinical usage of honey as a wound dressing: an update. *J Wound Care* **13**(9): 353–6

Moore O, Smith L, Campbell F, Seers K, McQuay H, Moore RA (2001) Systematic review of the use of honey as a wound dressing. *BMC Complementary and Alternative Medicine* **1**: 2

National Honey Board (2002) *Honey — Health and Therapeutic Qualities.* National Honey Board, USA

Postmes T, Bogaard A (1993) honey for wounds, ulcers, and skin graft preservation. *Lancet* **341**(8847): 756–7

Subrahmanyam M (1998) A prospective randomised clinical and histological study of superficial burn wound healing with honey and silver sulphadiazine. *Burns* **24**(2): 157–61

Tonks A, Cooper R, Price AP, Jones , Blair S, Parton J (2003) Honey stimulates inflammatory cytokine production from monocytes. *Cytokines* **21**: 242–7

Walsh J, Fairley J (1995) Calcifying diseases of the skin. *J Am Acad Dermatol* **33**: 693–706

Chapter 9

A summary of published clinical research on honey in wound management

Richard White and Peter Molan

This chapter is intended to provide a broad overview of the current clinical data published on honey in wound management. It is not presented as a review, systematic or otherwise. Whilst honey and honey-based treatments have been used on wounds for millennia, it is only recently that we have seen any attempt to provide meaningful clinical data on medical grade honey products. This is not to discount all previous data, as that does have a role in guidance. According to Molan (2002):

> *Dressing wounds with honey, a standard practice in past times, went out of fashion when antibiotics came into use. Because antibiotic-resistant bacteria have become a widespread clinical problem, a renaissance in honey use has occurred.*

In the past two decades, numerous laboratory studies and clinical trials have shown that honey is an effective broad-spectrum antibacterial agent that has no known adverse effects on wound tissues.

Clinically, topical honey treatment has been shown to have many key actions:

- antibacterial and antimicrobial
- autolytic debridement
- deodorises wounds
- stimulates growth of wound tissues to hasten healing and to start the healing process in dormant wounds
- anti-inflammatory activity rapidly reduces pain, oedema, and exudate and minimises hypertrophic scarring
- moist wound healing.

When looking at clinical evidence it is important to rank the available information according to current standards, thus a randomised clinical trial (RCT) is recognised as the highest level of clinical evidence. Such trials are very expensive in terms of time to plan, conduct, analyse and report, and, in terms of financial costs. However, this should not, and does not, discount all other evidence (Rolfe, 1999). A systematic review has been conducted on the published evidence on honey in wound care (Moore et al, 2001). This concluded that the evidence available (at that time) from seven comparative studies on 264 patients was limited by lack of 'blinding', poor reporting and poor validity. Much has changed since the Moore review; quality comparative studies have been set up and preliminary data reported on the new generation of 'Medical Device grade' honey products.

Until very recently, the honey used in wound management has been generic, non-sterile material, sourced from supplies intended for nutritional rather than medical use. However, in recent years, we have seen a number of honey-based wound treatments come to the UK market with the European Conformity (CE) mark and regulatory approval as sterile Medical Devices for use on full-thickness wounds (NZX, 2005).

Clinical reports

The topical application of honey has been reported to rapidly clear existing wound infection (Cavanagh et al, 1970; Efem, 1988 and 1993; Phuapradit and Saropala, 1992; Armon, 1980; Sofka et al, 2004): to facilitate healing of deeply infected surgical wounds (McInerey, 1990; Vardi et al, 1998; Al-Waili and Saloom, 1999; Cooper et al, 2001; Ahmed et al, 2003): and, halt spreading necrotising fasciitis (Hejase et al, 1996). In some cases, the application of honey has promoted healing in infected wounds that were not responding to conventional therapy (such as antibiotics and antiseptics: Wood et al, 1997; Harris, 1994; Dunford et al, 2000a,b; Ahmed et al, 2003) including wounds infected with antibiotic-resistant bacteria such as methicillin-resistant *Staphylococcus aureus* (Natarajan et al, 2001; Dunford et al, 2000; see *Chapter 2* for details of antibacterial activity). Honey rapidly deodorises wounds (Molan, 2002; Subrahmanyam, 1991; Kingsley, 2001; van der Weyden, 2003; Stephen-Haynes, 2004) and promotes autolytic debridement to facilitate the rapid development of a clean, granulating wound bed (Subhramanyam, 1998; Stephen-Haynes, 2004). A rapid rate of healing has been reported in wounds treated with honey (Hejase *et al,* 1996; Blomfield, 1973; Ahmed *et al,* 2003); this also serves to kick-start the healing process in otherwise 'dormant' wounds (Efem, 1988; Wood *et al,* 1997; Somerfield, 1991; Bloomfield, 1976; Stephen-Haynes, 2004). Also, honey has been reported to stimulate the growth of epithelium (Efem, 1993; Hejase *et al,* 1996; Subrahmanyam, 1994 and 1998), thus occasionally making plastic surgery unnecessary (Molan, 2001). It also is reported to minimise scarring (Efem 1993; Dunford *et al,* 2000a; Subrahmanyam, 1993 and 1994; Molan, 2001).

Honey reduces inflammation (Subrahmanyam 1998), oedema and exudate levels (Efem, 1993 and 1988; Hejase, *et al* 1996) and can have a 'soothing' effect when applied to wounds, including burns (Subrahmanyam 1993; Keast-Butler 1980) and donor sites (Misirlioglu *et al* 2003). However, some patients report a stinging sensation upon application (Vandeputte and Van Waeyenberge, 2003: see *Chapter 1*, and Table *10.1*).

Table 10.1: Reported pain on application of honey in a study of eighty-nine patients (from Vandeputte, 2003)

Wound type	No pain	Mild pain	Severe pain
Venous ulcers	31	4	1
Burns*	5	2	0
DFU	5	1	0
Mixed	9	2	3
Pressure ulcers	15	3	0
Skin tears	8	0	0

*Note: not all medical honey dressings are advocated for the treatment of full-thickness burns, always read the manufacturer's instructions before use.

In addition, honey has been used successfully on skin grafts, infected skin graft donor sites (Misirlioglu *et al,* 2003), infected traumatic wounds (Green 1988) and paediatric oncological lesions (Sofka *et al* 2004), necrotising fasciitis (or Fournier's gangrene: Hejase *et al,* 1996) abscesses, pilonidal sinuses, pressure ulcers, leg ulcers, diabetic ulcers (Tovey, 1991), tropical ulcers, sickle cell ulcers, and malignant ulcers (Efem, 1988).

Honey is also claimed to be a reliable alternative to conventional dressing for managing skin excoriation around stomas (ileostomy and colostomy), and facilitating epithelialisation of the damaged surface (Aminu _et al,_ 2000). This aspect of skin care is supported by reports of the beneficial effects of honey on paediatric (napkin/diaper) dermatitis (Al-Waili, 2005), and on atopic eczema and psoriasis (Al-Waili, 2003).

Comparative effectiveness

In three prospective, randomised, controlled clinical trials, honey was found to help heal superficial burns quicker than polyurethane film (OpSite™, Smith and Nephew), a dressing commonly used for providing a moist healing environment; and quicker than silver sulfadiazine (SSD) 1% ointment, the current 'gold standard' dressing for preventing infection in burn wounds (Pruitt, 1987). In a study comparing honey-impregnated gauze with the polyurethane film, the mean times to healing in each group (n = 46) were 10.8 days and 15.3 days respectively (p<0.001). In addition, significantly fewer honey-dressed wounds became infected (p<0.001; Subrahmanyam, 1993). In the first of the two studies that compared honey-impregnated gauze with silver sulfadiazine-impregnated gauze (n – 52 patients in each group), 87% of the wounds treated with honey healed within fifteen days, compared with 10% of those treated with SSD (p<0.001; Subrahmanyam 1991). In this study, a statistically significant difference (p<0.001) was found in the clearance of bacteria from the burns. In the forty-three out of fifty-two cases that presented positive swab cultures on admission in the group treated with honey, thirty-nine (91%) became sterile within seven days. In the comparison (SSD) group, only three (7%) of forty-one wounds with positive swab cultures became sterile: evidence of the antibacterial effect of honey _in vivo._

In the second burns trial (twenty-five patients in each group), 100% of the wounds treated with honey healed within twenty-one days, compared to twenty-one (84%) of those treated with SSD (p<0.001; Subrahmanyam, 1998). In addition to the significant difference found in burn wound healing, biopsies of the treated areas showed greater histopathological evidence of reparative activity. This was seen in 80% of wounds treated with honey dressing compared to 52% of the wounds treated with SSD (p<0.005; noted in biopsy samples from the wound margins after seven days of treatment). Regarding the clearance of bacteria from burns, in twenty-three of the twenty-five cases treated with honey that had positive swab cultures on admission in the group, fifteen (65%) of the wounds became sterile in seven days and twenty-two (96%) in twenty-one days. By comparison, of the twenty-two wounds with positive cultures treated with SSD, sixteen (73%) became sterile in seven days, and nineteen (86%) in twenty-one days (p<0.001). This is further evidence of the antibacterial effect of honey *in vivo*.

Although these trials showed that honey offered better control of infection than standard treatment, a trial on moderate burns where half of the total burn area was full-thickness showed that control of infection was better with early tangential excision followed with autologous skin grafting than with honey treatment (Subrahmanyam, 1999). In two groups (n = 25) of young adults, 34% of swab cultures were positive for the group treated with honey, compared with 10% of the group treated with early tangential excision (p<0.05). Antibiotics were needed for 32±18 days in the honey-treated group compared with 16±3 days in the excision group (p<0.001). These findings relate to the need to debride eschar as it serves as a 'reservoir' of potential pathogens in the burn. The mean blood volume replaced was less with the honey treatment (21% ± 15%, compared with 35% ± 12%, p<0.01) and skin grafting was required on only eleven patients of the group treated with honey.

In recent reports where selected honey was used on an infected wound following surgical treatment of hidradenitis suppurativa (Cooper *et al,* 2001) and infected skin lesions from meningococcal septicaemia (Dunford, 2000a), the antibacterial activity gave rise to rapid clearance of infection and healing of the wounds. In both of these studies, it had not been possible to achieve healing with the many systemic antibiotics and modern dressing materials previously tried over a long period of time. Good infection control was reported in a crossover study of nine infants with large infected surgical wounds (Vardi, 1998). Honey was used on the wounds after they failed to heal following at least fourteen days of treatments with intravenous antibiotics (a combination of vancomycin and cefotaxime, subsequently changed according to bacterial sensitivity), fusidic acid ointment, and wound cleaning with aqueous 0.05% chlorhexidine solution. Marked clinical improvement was seen in all cases after five days of treatment; all wounds were closed, clean, and sterile after twenty-one days of honey application. A prospective, randomised controlled trial on severe post-operative wound infections following caesarean section or abdominal hysterectomy was conducted to compare dressing with honey (n = 26) to washing wounds with 70%

ethanol and applying povidone-iodine (n = 24). Both groups received systemic antibiotics according to culture and sensitivity. In the group treated with honey, infection was rapidly eradicated (6±1.9 days vs 14.8±4.2 days), wounds healed faster (10.7±2.5 days vs 22±7.3 days), post-operative scars were less than half the size, and the period of hospitalisation was less than half of that for the patients in the control group (9.4±1.8 days vs 19.9±7.4 days: p<0.05 for each parameter: Al-Waili and Saloom, 1999). This study was of particular interest as all patients were treated with appropriate antibiotics, yet the topical application of honey still proved to be effective in reducing bioburden. This might be due to low local tissue levels of antibiotic from poor perfusion of the wound. It is of interest that _in vitro_ studies have shown a synergy between honey and common antibiotics in multidrug resistant _Pseudomonas spp_ (Karayil _et al_, 1998). It would, therefore, appear to justify the combination of systemic antibiotics with use of topical antibacterials (such as honey) in wounds where poor perfusion and drug resistance might compromise healing.

A trial on patients with dehisced abdominal wounds following caesarean section, showed healing in less than half the time (mean length of stay in hospital 4.5 days, range two to seven days) when the wound was dressed with honey, compared retrospectively with the usual treatment of wound care (cleansing with hydrogen peroxide solution, Dakin's solution, and packing with saline-soaked gauze) and subsequent re-suturing (mean length of stay in hospital 11.5 days, range nine to eighteen days: Phuapradit and Saropala, 1992).

Wound deodorising

Malodour is a common feature of chronic wounds; it is attributed to the presence of anaerobic bacterial species such as _Bacteroides spp_, _Peptostreptococci_ and _Prevotella spp_ (Bowler _et al_, 1999). It is probably more than just the antibacterial action that is responsible for the rapid deodorising of wounds observed when honey dressings are used. The malodorous substances produced by bacteria are short-chain fatty acids, ammonia, amines, and sulphur compounds. These are formed by the metabolism of amino acids from decomposed serum and tissue proteins. Honey provides a copious quantity of glucose, a substrate metabolised by bacteria in preference to amino acids.

Immune system activity

The clearance of infection may not only be the result of the antibacterial action of honey. Recent research indicates that honey may work by stimulating the activity of the immune system. Honey at concentrations as low as 0.1% has been found to stimulate proliferation of peripheral blood β-lymphocytes and T-lymphocytes in cell culture and activate phagocytes from blood. Also, honey at a concentration of 1% has been reported to stimulate monocytes in cell culture to release the cytokines TNF-1, IL-1, and IL-6, which are intermediates in the immune response. In addition to the reported stimulation of leukocytes, honey has the potential to augment further the immune response by supplying glucose. This is essential for the 'respiratory burst' in macrophages that generates hydrogen peroxide, the dominant component of the bacteria-destroying activity of these cells (see Molan, 2002).

Wound debridement

Like any other moist wound dressing, honey facilitates the debridement of wounds by the autolytic action of tissue proteases. Unlike other wound dressings, honey creates a moist environment by drawing out lymph fluid from the wound tissues through its strong osmotic action. This provides a constantly replenished supply of proteases at the interface of the wound bed and the overlying necrotic tissue, which may, in part, explain the rapid debridement brought about by honey. This osmotic action also washes the surface of the wound bed from beneath. This explains the frequent observation of honey dressings removing debris such as foreign bodies (eg. dirt, grit) with the dressing (Molan, 2002). It also helps explain the painless lifting off of slough and necrotic tissue that is observed (Efem, 1988 and 1993; Hejase *et al*, 1996; Subrahmanyam, 1993 and 1998). Another possible explanation for the observed rapid debridement is activation of the proteases by hydrogen peroxide liberated by honey. The proteases in wound tissues are normally in an inactive state but can be activated by oxidation. The matrix metalloproteases of connective tissue, normally present in a catalytically inactive conformation, may be activated by the hydrogen peroxide (Peppin and Weiss, 1986; Weiss *et al*, 1985). High protease activity is strongly associated with impaired wound healing, which may suggest that activation of proteases by honey would be harmful rather than beneficial. However, a causal effect has never been proved (Ashcroft et al, 2000); possibly, the association is the result of both impaired healing and high protease activity together caused by the same factor — excessive, uncontrolled inflammation (Agren et al, 2000). Excessive inflammation prevents healing and the attraction of inflammatory leukocytes gives rise to high levels of proteolytic enzyme activity at the site of the inflammation (Ashcroft et al, 2000; Agren et al, 2000). The potent anti-inflammatory action of honey (see below) would resolve such a situation and prevent excessive proteolytic activity. It also has been suggested that high levels of proteolytic activity and high levels of inflammation are both caused by a lack of secretory leukocyte protease inhibitor, which is an inhibitor both of serine proteases and the production of TGF-β, a potent chemoattractant of inflammatory cells. Yet, proteolysis in wound tissues is a normal part of the healing process and responsible for autolytic debridement.

Anti-inflammatory action

Clinical observations of reduced inflammation following application of honey to a wound are substantiated by the results of _in vivo_ studies that have shown that honey, when compared to various controls, reduces inflammation. Histological evidence of reduced numbers of inflammatory cells present in wounds dressed with honey exists from studies of deep (Postmes et al, 1997) and superficial burns, as well as full-thickness wounds. These effects were due to components other than the sugar in honey (Postmes et al, 1997). Evidence also has come from similar findings in biopsy samples from burn wound tissue of hospital patients (Subrahmanyam, 1998). Although it is a vital part of the normal response to infection or injury, excessive or prolonged inflammation can prevent healing or even cause further damage to tissues (Agren et al, 2000). Suppressing inflammation, as well as reducing pain for the patient, reduces the opening of blood vessels, thus reducing oedema and exudate. Pressure in tissues secondary to oedema restricts the flow of blood through the capillaries, starving the tissues of the oxygen and the nutrients vital for leukocytes to fight infection and for fibroblasts to multiply for wound healing. Finally, healing may be impaired because swelling increases the distance for diffusion of oxygen and nutrients from the capillaries to the cells.

Stimulation of tissue growth

The evidence provided supports the following statements:

* Honey is a bioactive wound dressing that provides rapid wound healing.
* Honey promotes the formation of clean healthy granulation tissue and re-epithelialisation.
* The stimulation of cell growth seen with honey is probably also responsible for 'kick-starting' the healing process in chronic wounds that have remained non-healing for long periods.

Conclusions

The clinical evidence for the use of honey in wound management is steadily accumulating and, with the advent of various forms of manufactured honey dressings currently commercially available or being developed for marketing, the flow of evidence will continue. Whilst the evidence pre-2000 was on generic honeys, more recent research has been focused on the sterile medical grade honey products intended specifically for wound management. These products have been designed to overcome many of the problems of messiness and difficulty of handling, making honey-based products as convenient to use as the more familiar modern wound dressings. Some involve the combination of honey with a modern dressing such as alginate or sheet hydrogel. Others present honey as a tubed formulation of amorphous gel or of ointment. This brings the most ancient form of wound dressing known into the realms of the most modern — an easy-to-use, bioactive dressing that provides a moist healing environment, with the advantage of having within a single product a range of actions (debriding, deodorising, antibacterial, growth-promoting, anti-inflammatory, and scar-minimising), usually available only individually in a range of products. These attributes will, no doubt, be shown to be cost-effective in future clinical research.

References _____

Agren MS, Eaglstein WH, Ferguson MW *et al* (2000) Causes and effects of the chronic inflammation in venous leg ulcers. *Acta Derm Venereol* (Stockh) **210**: 3–17

Ahmed AK, Hoekstra MJ, Hage J, Karim RB (2003) Honey-medicated dressing: transformation of an ancient remedy into modern therapy. *Ann Plast Surg* **50**(2): 143–8

Al-Waili NS, Saloom KY (1999) Effects of topical honey on post-operative wound infections due to Gram positive and Gram negative bacteria following caesarean sections and hysterectomies. *Eur J Med Res* **4**: 126–30

Al-Waili NS (2005) Clinical and mycological benefits of topical application of honey, olive oil and beeswax in diaper dermatitis. *Clin Microbiol Inf Dis* **11**(2): 160–3

Al-Waili NS (2003) Topical application of natural honey, beeswax and olive oil mixture to treat patients with atopic dermatitis or psoriasis: partially controlled study *Complement Ther Med* **11**: 222–6

Aminu SR, Hassan AW, Babayo U (2000) Another use of honey. *Trop Doct* **30**(4): 250–1

Armon PJ (1980) The use of honey in the treatment of infected wounds. *Trop Doct* **10**: 91

Ashcroft GS, Lei K, Jin W *et al* (2000) Secretory leucocyte protease inhibitor mediates non-redundant functions necessary for normal wound healing. *Nat Med* **6**(10): 1147–53

Bloomfield E (1976) Old remedies. *Br J Gen Pract* **26**: 576

Blomfield R (1973) Honey for decubitus ulcers. *JAMA* **224**(6): 905

Bowler PG, Davies BJ, Jones SA (1999) Microbial involvement in chronic wound malodour. *J Wound Care* **8**(5): 216–8

Braniki FJ (1981) Surgery in Western Kenya. *Ann R Coll Surg Engl* **63**: 348–52

Cavanagh D, Beazley J, Ostapowicz F (1970) Radical operation for carcinoma of the vulva. A new approach to wound healing. *J Obstet Gynaecol Br Commonwealth* **77**(11): 1037–40

Chant A (1999) The biomechanics of leg ulceration. *Ann R Coll Surg Engl* **81**: 80–5

Chung LY, Schmidt RJ, Andrews AM, Turner TD (1993) A study of hydrogen peroxide generation by, and antioxidant activity of Granuflex Hydrocolloid Granules and some other hydrogel/hydrocolloid wound management materials. *Br J Dermatol* **129**(2): 145–53

Cooper RA, Molan PC (1999) The use of honey as an antiseptic in managing *Pseudomonas* infection. *J Wound Care* **8**(4): 161–4

Cooper RA, Molan PC, Harding KG (1999) Antibacterial activity of honey against strains of *Staphylococcus aureus* from infected wounds. *J R Soc Med* **92**: 283–5

Cooper RA, Molan PC, Krishnamoorthy L, Harding K (2001) Manuka honey used to heal a recalcitrant surgical wound. *Eur J Clin Microbiol Infect Dis* **20**: 858–759

Dunford C, Cooper RA, Molan PC (2000) Using honey as a dressing for infected skin lesions. *Nurs Times* **96**(14) (NT Plus): 7–9

Dunford C, Cooper RA, White RJ, Molan PC (2000) The use of honey in wound management. *Nurs Standard* **15**(11): 63–8

Efem SEE (1993) Recent advances in the management of Fournier's gangrene: preliminary observations. *Surgery* **113**(2): 200–4

Efem SEE (1988) Clinical observations on the wound healing properties of honey. *Br J Surg* **75**: 679–81

Green AE (1988) Wound healing properties of honey. *Br J Surg* **75**(12): 1278

Harris S (1994) Honey for the treatment of superficial wounds: a case report and review. *Primary Intention* **2**(4): 18–23

Jones HR (2001) Honey and healing through the ages. In: Munn PA, Jones HR, eds. *Honey and Healing*. IBRA, Cardiff, UK: 1–4

Karayil S, Deshpande SD, Koppikar GV (1998) Effect of honey on multidrug resistant organisms and its synergistic action with three common antibiotics. *J Postgrad Med* **44**(4): 93–6

Kaufman T, Eichenlaub EH, Angel MF *et al* (1985) Topical acidification promotes healing of experimental deep partial-thickness skin burns: a randomised double-blind preliminary study. *Burns* **12**: 84–90

Keast-Butler J (1980) Honey for necrotic malignant breast ulcers. *Lancet* **ii**: 809

Kingsley AR (2001) The use of honey in the treatment of infected wounds: case studies. *Br J Nurs* **10**(22) (suppl): s13–s20

Lawrence JC (1999) Editorial: Honey and wound bacteria. *J Wound Care* **8**(4): 155

Misirlioglu A, Eroglu S *et al* (2003) Use of honey as an adjunct in the healing of split-thickness skin graft donor sites. *Dermatol Surg* **29**(2): 168–72

McInerney RJF (1990) Honey — a remedy rediscovered. *J R Soc Med* **83**: 127

Molan PC (1998) A brief review of honey as a clinical dressing. *Primary Intention* **6**(4): 148–58

Molan PC (2001) Potential of honey in the treatment of wounds and burns. *Am J Clin Dermatol* **2**(1): 13–9

Molan PC (2002) Re-introducing honey in the management of wounds and ulcers — theory and practice. *Ostomy Wound Manag* **48**(11): 28–40

Moore OA, Smith LA, Campbell F *et al* (2001) Systematic review of honey as a wound dressing. *BMC Complem Alt Med* **1**(2): 1

Natarajan S, Williamson D, Grey J, Harding KG, Cooper RA (2001) Healing of an MRSA-colonized hydroxyurea induced leg ulcer with honey. *J Dermatol Treat* **12**: 33–6

Nielsen ER (1991) *Honey in Medicine*. VI Congresso Internationale di Egottologia (Atti). Turin: 415–9

NZX (2005) New Zealand Stock Exchange report www.nzx.com/market

Peppin GJ, Weiss SJ (1986) Activation of the endogenous metalloproteinase, gelatinase, by triggered human neutrophils. *Proc Natl Acad Sci USA* **83**: 4322–26

Phuapradit W, Saropala N (1992) Topical application of honey in treatment of abdominal wound disruption. *Aust N Z J Obstet Gynaecol* **32**(4): 381–4

Potmes TJ, Bosch MMC *et al* (1997) Speeding up the healing of burns with honey. An experimental study with histological assessment of wound biopsies. In: Mizrahi A, lensky Y, eds. *Bee Products: Properties, applications and apitherapy*. Plenum Press, New York: 27–37

Postmes T, Vandeputte J (1999) Recombinant growth factors or honey? *Burns* **25**(7): 676–78

Pruitt BA (1987) Opportunistic infections in burns patients. In: Root R, Trunkey R, Sande MA, eds. *New Surgical Approaches to Infectious Diseases*. Churchill Livingstone, New York. 245–61

Rolfe G (1999) Insufficient evidence: the problem of evidence-based nursing. *Nurs Educ Today* **19**(6): 433–42

Root-Bernstein R, Root-Bernstein M (1999) *Honey, Mud, Maggots and other Medical Marvels*. Macmillan, London

Silvetti AN (1981) An effective method of treating long-enduring wounds and ulcers by topical applications of solutions of nutrients. *J Dermatol Surg Oncol* **7**(6): 501–8

Sinclair RD, Ryan TJ (1994) Proteolytic enzymes in wound healing: the role of enzymatic debridement. *Aust J Dermatol* **35**: 35–41

Sofka K, Wisznewsky G Blaser G *et al* (2004) Antibakterieller Honig (Medihoney) zur Wundpflege-Wundantisepsis bei patiatrischen Patienten in der Hamatologie-Onkologie? *Krankenhaus Hygiene + Infektion verhutung* **26**(5): 183–7

Somerfield SD (1991) Honey and healing. *J R Soc Med* **84**(3): 179

Stephen-Haynes (2004) Evaluation of honey-impregnated tulle dressing in primary care. *Br J Community Nurs* **9**(6) (suppl): s21–s27

Subrahmanyam M (1991) Topical application of honey in treatment of burns. *Br J Surg* **78**(4): 497–8

Subrahmanyam M (1993) Honey-impregnated gauze versus polyurethane film (OpSite) in the treatment of burns — a prospective randomised study. *Br J Plast Surg* **46**(4): 322–3

Subrahmanyam M (1994) Honey-impregnated gauze versus amniotic membrane in the treatment of burns. *Burns* **20**(44): 331–3

Subrahmanyam M (1996) Honey dressing versus boiled potato peel in the treatment of burns: a prospective randomized study. *Burns* **22**(6): 491–3

Subrahmanyam M (1998) A prospective randomised clinical and histological study of superficial burn wound healing with honey and silver sulfadiazine. *Burns* **24**(2): 157–61

Subrahmanyam M (1999) Early tangential excision and skin grafting of moderate burns is superior to honey dressing: a prospective randomised trial. *Burns* **25**(8): 729–31

Subrahmanyam M, Ugane SP (2004) Honey dressing beneficial in treatment of Fournier's gangrene. *Ind J Surg* **66**(2): 75–7

Tovey FL (1991) Honey and healing. *J R Soc Med* **84**(7): 447

van der Weyden E (2003) The use of honey for the treatment of two patients with pressure ulcers. *Br J Community Nurs* **8**(12) (suppl): s14–s20

Weiss SJ, Peppin G *et al* (1985) Oxidative autoactivation of latent collagenase by human neutrophils. *Science* **227**: 747–9

Willix DJ, Molan PC, Harfoot CJ (1992) A comparison of the sensitivity of wound-infecting species of bacteria to the antibacterial activity of Manuka honey and other honey. *J Appl Bacteriol* **73**: 388–94

Vandeputte J, Van Waeyenberge PH (2003) Clinical evaluation of L-Mesitran, a honey-based wound ointment. *EWMA J* **3**(2): 8–11

Vardi A, Barzilay Z, Linder N, Cohen HA, Paret G (1998) Local application of honey for treatment of neonatal postoperative wound infection. *Acta Paediatr* **87**(4): 429–32

Wood B, Rademaker M, Molan PC (1997) Manuka honey, a low cost leg ulcer dressing. *N Z Med J* **110**: 107

Zumla A, Lulat A (1989) Honey — a remedy rediscovered. *J R Soc Med* **82**: 384–5

CHAPTER 10

IMMUNOMODULATORY PROPERTIES OF HONEY THAT MAY BE RELEVANT TO WOUND REPAIR

Rose Cooper, Ken Jones and Keith Morris

Wound healing is a complex process that involves both a degenerative and reparative phase (Clarke, 1996). The tissue macrophages are cells that are crucial in regulating wound healing. Macrophages are cells derived from peripheral blood monocytes; their role involves:

- the removal of damaged connective tissue and cell debris resulting from infection or injury
- the killing and removal pathogens
- the formation of new blood vessels
- the stimulation of fibroblast proliferation that results in collagen biosynthesis that gives rise to the remodelling of connective tissue.

Macrophages are capable of synthesising and secreting cytokines, important molecules that modulate the immune response. These include Tumour Necrosis Factor-α (TNF-α). Macrophages produce reactive intermediates (ROIs) and hydrolytic enzymes that are involved in microbial killing. They also produce growth factors and vasoactive agents which promote the repair process, attract cells to the site of tissue damage eventually leading to the removal of dead or damaged cells and tissue (Jones, 2001).

The antimicrobial and anti-inflammatory properties of honey are well established (Molan, 1999). The ability of Manuka, jellybush and pasture honey to stimulate monocytes, the precursors of macrophages, to secrete TNF-α has been investigated (Tonks *et al*, 2001; Tonks *et al*, 2003). The honeys were able to increase significantly the secretion of TNF-α

and other cytokines by monocytes. The honey samples, tested as being endotoxin free, were added to cell cultures as 1% (w/v) solutions and incubated for twenty-four hours. Activation of these cells may, in part, explain the well-documented wound healing qualities of honeys such as these. Honey has the potential to aid wound healing by the ability of its glycosylated proteins or other components to stimulate cytokines such as TNF-α by macrophages. Glycosylated proteins are known to induce TNF-α secretion by macrophages, and this cytokine is known to induce wound repair mechanisms. Furthermore, the ability of honey to reduce ROI release (Tonks *et al*, 2001) may well limit tissue damage by activated macrophages during wound healing. Leakage of these components from activated cells is responsible for much of the damage to tissue that is seen after infection and tissue damage. Kasri (2004) has shown that blocking Toll-like Receptor 4 (Toll receptor: one of a family of receptors that provide a critical link between immune stimulants produced by micro-organisms and the initiation of the host defence; TLR 4 binds lipopolysaccharide LPS. Activation of the toll receptors causes the release of antimicrobial peptides, inflammatory cytokines, and molecules that initiate adaptive immunity) diminished, but did not prevent, TNF-α synthesis in monocytes.

An inference from this observation is that TNF-α release from monocytes may be elicited by more than one factor.

Inflammation is part of the normal response to infection and wounding and inflammatory signals, such as lipopolysaccharide (or endotoxin), can induce release of prostaglandin E_2 (PGE$_2$) from monocytes and macrophages via cyclo-oxygenase$_2$ metabolism. PGE$_2$ modulates several inflammatory responses, increases vascular permeability and sensitivity to pain, as well as being pyrogenic. There are reports that some patients find honey soothing, but that others experience a stinging sensation. Although Al-Waili and Boni (2003) have demonstrated lowered plasma prostaglandin levels in normal individuals following oral administration of honey, a recent study (similar to Tonks *et al*, 2001, and 2003), showed that Manuka honey was able to increase significantly prostaglandin E_2 synthesis in monocytic cells (Morris *et al*, 2004). PGE$_2$ has been shown to be an important component in regulating wound repair in keratinocytes (Rys-Sikora *et al*, 2000).

Of the numerous cytokines produced at wound sites, the transforming growth factor-beta (TGF-β) superfamily has the most profound ability to influence many aspects of tissue repair. The three main isoforms (TGF β_1, $_2$, and $_3$) have all been localised in healing wounds. The manipulation of the ratios, particularly of β_1 relative to β_3, reduces scarring and fibrosis

(O'Kane and Ferguson, 1997). TGF-β is released by degranulating platelets, and secreted by lymphocytes, macrophages, endothelial cells, smooth muscle cells, epithelial cells and fibroblasts (Roberts and Sporn, 1996). Human cells produce all three isoforms, of which TGF-α_1 is best-studied (Philipp *et al*, 2004). The importance of TGF-α_1 in wound healing has been reviewed (Kim *et al*, 2005). There is currently limited evidence as to the ability of honey to regulate TGF-α_1 synthesis. In a recent study, propolis, the resinous product collected by honey bees from plants that has been used in folk medicine since ancient times, has been shown to be able to increase TGF-α_1 secretion by immune cells (Ansorge *et al*, 2003).

Advances in understanding the mechanisms of wound healing are of great importance in developing appropriate strategies for the clinical management of wounds. In this respect, the nuclear receptor peroxisome proliferator-activated receptor (PPAR)-β/δ occupies a unique position at the intersection of the pro-inflammatory and anti-inflammatory signals important in wound repair (Tan *et al*, 2005). The precise function of PPAR-β/δ is as yet not fully elucidated, although it is known to have a critical role in the response of keratinocytes to the inflammatory signals produced after skin injury. Although fatty acids can bind and activate PPAR-β/δ, studies on this isotype have so far been impeded by the lack of information about the nature of its physiological ligands and by its remarkably broad tissue distribution. The inflammation that immediately follows injury increases the expression of PPAR-β/δ in the wound edge keratinocytes, and triggers the production of endogenous PPAR-β/δ ligands that activate the newly produced receptor. This elevated PPAR-β/δ activity results in increased resistance of the keratinocytes to the apoptotic signals released during wounding, allowing faster re epithelialisation.

Changes in PPAR-β/δ expression can have a profound effect on wound healing, and, as shown in a recent study (Tan *et al*, 2005), dictate wound repair kinetics. Following topical application of TGF-β_1 to skin wounds, a crucial dual role of TGF-β_1 as a chemoattractant of inflammatory cells and repressor of inflammation-induced PPAR-β/δ expression, was revealed.

The immediate response to trauma in the skin is the release of inflammatory signals. In a study (Tan *et al*, 2001) which used cultured or primary keratinocytes from wild-type and PPAR-β/δ^{--} mice, that such signals including TNF-α and IFN-γ, induce keratinocyte differentiation was demonstrated. This cytokine-dependent cell differentiation pathway requires up-regulation of the PPAR-β/δ gene via the stress-associated kinase cascade, which targets a receptor on the PPAR-β/δ promoter. In addition, pro-inflammatory cytokines, such as TNF-α, also initiate the production of endogenous PPAR-β/δ ligands, which are essential for PPAR-β/δ activation and action. Activated PPAR-β/δ regulates the expression of genes associated with apoptosis, resulting in an increased resistance of keratinocytes to cell death. This effect is also observed *in vivo* during wound healing after an injury. Recent, unpublished results from our laboratory has demonstrated that Manuka honey is capable of significantly increasing the expression of PPAR-β/δ in human monocytes. Although this result as yet remains unconfirmed in keratinocytes it is, nevertheless, early evidence that honey may induce expression of this important nuclear receptor involved in wound repair.

The provision of nutrients that enhance cell growth is another way that honey may stimulate healing in chronic wounds. A recent study has indicated that glucose enhanced the proliferation of human dermal fibroblasts *in vitro* (Hanet *et al*, 2004). Since glucose levels in exudates collected from chronic wounds are low (Trengove *et al*, 1996), and honey contains approximately 33.5% glucose, it is possible that topical application of honey to chronic wounds helps to promote local cell growth.

There is one laboratory observation that helps to explain the documented clinical benefits of honey as a debriding agent. Proteolytic activity of honey from two different species of bees has been measured in bovine fibrinogen, with maximum activity at pH 5–6 (Oliveira *et al*, 2004). Previously, hydrolytic activity had not been associated with honey.

Conclusion

The evidence that honey has an increasingly important role in wound repair will involve studies that investigate its ability to both modulate and interact with nuclear receptors such as PPAR-β/δ, and to release cytokines such as TNF-α and TGF-α_1. The complexity and variety of the components present in honey, requires a greater understanding of how they act, both individually and collectively, before deductions about specific mechanisms and clinical effects are possible.

References

Al-Waili NS, Boni NS (2003) Natural honey lowers plasma prostaglandin concentrations in normal individuals. _J Med Food_ **6**(2): 129–33

Ansorge S, Reinhold D, Lendeckel U (2003) Propolis and some of its constituents down-regulate DNA synthesis and inflammatory cytokine production but induce TGF-β_1 production of human immune cells. _Z Naturforsch_ **58**: 580–9

Clarke RAF (1996) Wound repair. In: Clarke RAF, ed. _The Molecular and Cellular Biology of Wound Repair_. 2nd edn. Plenum Press, New York: 3–50

Han J, Hughes MA, Cherry GW (2004) Effect of glucose concentration on the growth of normal human dermal fibroblasts in vitro. _J Wound Care_ **13**(4): 150–3

Jones KP (2000) The role of honey in wound healing and repair. In: Munn P, Jones R, eds. _Honey and Healing_. IBRA, Cardiff, UK

Kasri SS (2004) Investigating the immune stimulatory activity of honey. MSc thesis. University of Wales Institute, Cardiff, UK

Kim IY, Kim MM, Kim SJ (2005) Transforming growth factor-beta: biology and clinical relevance. _J Biochem Mol Biol_ **38**(1): 1–8

Molan PC (1999) The role of honey in the management of wounds. _J Wound Care_ **8**: 415–18

Morris RHK, Al-Balushi O, Cooper RA (2004) Manuka honey upregulates prostaglandin E_2 production in human monocytes. Poster presentation at 8th IBRA International Conference on Tropical Bees. Ribeirao Preto, Brazil

O'Kane S, Ferguson MW (1997) Transforming growth factor beta and wound healing. _Int J Biochem Cell Biol_ **29**(1): 63–78

Oliveira CC, Menezes C, Torres FS, Kerr WE, Oliveira F (2004) Proteolytic activity of honey from _Apis mellifera_ and _Tetragona clavipes_. Proc. 8th IBRA International Conference on Tropical Bees and VI Encontro sobre Abelhas. Ribeirao Preto, Brazil

Philipp K, Reidel F, Sauerbier M et al (2004) Targeting TGF-beta in human keratinocytes and its potential in wound healing. _Int J Mol Med_ **14**(4): 589–93

Roberts AR, Sporn MB (1996) Transforming growth factor-α. In: Clarke RAF, ed. _The Molecular and Cellular Biology of Wound Repair_. 2nd edn. Plenum Press, New York: 275–308

Rys-Sikora KE, Konger RL, Schoggins JW, Malaviya R, Pentland AP (2000) Coordinate expression of secretory phospholipase A(2) and cyclooxygenase-$_2$ in activated human keratinocytes. *Am J Physiol Cell Physiol* **278**(4): C822–33.

Tan NS, Michalik L, Noy N, Yasmin R, Pacot C, Heim M *et al* (2001) Critical roles of PPAR-β/δ in keratinocyte response to inflammation. *Genes Dev* **15**: 3263–77

Tan NS, Michalik L, Desvergne B, Wahli W (2005) Genetic- or TGF-β_1 induced changes in epidermal PPAR-β/δ expression dictate wound repair kinetics. *J Biol Chem* (in press). E-published ahead of print

Tonks AJ, Cooper RA, Jones KP, Blair S, Parton J, Tonks A (2003) Honey stimulates inflammatory cytokine production from monocytes. *Cytokine* **21**(5): 242–7

Tonks A, Cooper RA, Price AJ, Molan PC, Jones KP (2001) Stimulation of TNF-alpha release in monocytes by honey. *Cytokine* **14**(4): 240–2

Trengove NJ, Stanton SR, Stacey MC (1996) Biochemical analysis of wound fluid from non-healing and healing chronic leg ulcers. *Wound Rep Regen* **4**: 234–9

Appendix

Guidelines for the use of honey in wound management

Val Robson

For those readers, who, like the author, underwent nurse training in the early 1970s, the use of honey in wound management will not be a new concept. Two milestones have revolutionised the management of wounds. First, the introduction of antibiotics, and, second the work carried out by Winter in 1962 introducing the concept that a warm moist environment encouraged healing. However, Winter's research took some twenty years to come to a routine clinical fruition with the inception of dressings that would provide an ideal healing environment. It was during the intervening years that honey was regularly used alongside hydrogen peroxide, yoghurt, egg white and oxygen, all used to debride and encourage new cell growth in wounds healing by secondary intention. When one considers that one of the qualities of honey is its weak (dilute), but long-acting and effective hydrogen peroxide content, then maybe its use in wound care management should not be surprising.

In recent years honey has enjoyed a renaissance with considerable amounts of research being performed in New Zealand, Australia and the UK (Molan and Betts, 2004; Cooper and Molan, 1999; Molan 1999; Dunford and Hanano, 2004; Willix *et al*, 1992; Cooper *et al*, 1999) adding to an existing body of evidence. Even though honey has a long history of over 4000 years as a natural remedy in the field of wound care, it is only in comparatively recent years that it has caught media attention. This has catapulted honey into public awareness, resulting in many patients arriving in clinics armed with jars of honey and newspaper cuttings extolling its virtues. This led to the dilemma of patients being keen to experiment, while nurses felt that they would be stepping outside their role accountability if they were to apply a product to a wound that was not licensed for that purpose. This problem has now been resolved with the introduction to the UK Drug Tariff honey-based wound treatments that are regulated and sterilised by gamma radiation specifically for wound care. This method of sterilisation has no detrimental effects on the antibacterial quality of honey (Molan and Allen, 1996), but renders it safe from clostridial spores, which may cause wound botulism.

Honey provides a moist environment to promote healing and acts as a viscous barrier to minimise microbial invasion and fluid loss which, in turn, limits cross-infection (Molan, 1999). The antimicrobial quality of honey contributes to the rapid clearance of infection, the reduction of bacterial burden, and the elimination of odour (Molan, 1999). Honey is reported to act as a debriding agent, to be an anti-inflammatory and, therefore, prepares the wound bed to hasten healing (Molan, 1999). The constituents of honey and mode of action are covered in *Chapters 1 and 2*.

There will always be some wounds that fail to heal due to some patients' predisposing medical problems. Whilst there are a plethora of dressings designed to manage any wound at any stage of healing, the need for new and innovative ways of managing wounds will be required to aid wound healing. Non-healing wounds have substantial financial and social consequences for national and personal situations.

Wounds that fail to heal present the healthcare professional with a variety of problems that require individual attention, such as copious exudate, malodour and recurrent infections.

Classification of wounds suitable for treatment with honey

Chronic wounds

Chronic wounds fail to heal at predicted rates, and instead of transition from the acute inflammatory phase into the proliferative phase, a transition into chronic inflammation occurs (Cooper, 2001). This type of wound often accommodates areas of non-viable tissue, such as necrosis and slough, along with areas of healthy granulation and epithelialising tissue. Holistic assessment and the correct dressing selection are vital to remove the non-viable tissue and to encourage the fragile new tissue growth.

The evidence to underpin the ability of honey to deal with characteristics proven to delay healing are well documented (Dunford *et al*, 2000; Efem, 1988; Robson, 2004; Dunford, 2000; see *Chapter 9* for details).

Honey has been used successfully on:

- leg ulceration (Robson, 2003; Natarajan *et al*, 2001; Alcaraz and Kelly, 2002)
- abdominal wound disruption (Phuapradit and Saropala, 1992)
- burns (Subrahmanyam, 1994; Bowler *et al*, 1999)
- infected donor sites*
- chronic inflammation (Robson, 2004; Dunford, 2000)
- preparation of the wound bed for split skin grafting*
- sinus*
- radiation necrosis*

* unpublished work. Clinical observation by author.

Malodorous wounds

Wound odour is commonly due to the presence of both aerobic and anaerobic bacteria within the wound (Bowler *et al*, 1999). The resulting effect is either elevated bioburden of the wound, causing no overt reaction, or clinical infection, causing the host to display the clinical symptoms of infection, ie. pain, swelling, erythema and heat. Once the presence of micro-organisms has started to grow and divide and establish wound infection or colonisation, the wound healing process will be arrested and the risk of cross-infection increased. Wound infection is one of the most significant factors that delay healing, although there is currently no consensus on the impact of specific micro-organisms on the healing process (White *et al*, 2001).

There have been numerous reported cases of reduction or elimination of wound odour following the application of honey (Dunford and Hanano, 2004; Robson, 2003; Alcaraz and Kelly, 2002; Kingsley, 2001). Many patients presenting with chronic wounds find the odour from the wound the most difficult symptom to live with (*Chapter 8*). The consequence of this manifestation has adverse effects on their quality of life, social activities and family life. Following the application of honey, odour control is rapid, and, when combined with a necessary increase in the frequency of dressing renewal, this has a positive effect on both the wound and patient.

Acute wounds

Honey has been used successfully on donor and recipient sites. After harvesting, the honey is applied directly to the donor site with a non-adherent primary dressing. A secondary alginate dressing is applied to manage exudate. This dressing is changed after two days and honey and adhesive foam applied daily thereafter. It has been observed that exudate is quickly reduced and scarring is minimised. The recipient site has the perforated donor skin applied and then covered with Jelonet™ (Smith and Nephew). Jelonet is applied to any cavities within the wound and honey is applied with an alginate dressing to manage any exudate. A Surgipad™ (Johnson and Johnson) is then placed *in situ* with a wool and crepe bandage to secure. This dressing remains in place for five days. A new dressing of honey is applied to a non-adherent silicone dressing which is covered with a pad and secured with a wool and crepe. The procedure is repeated either daily or on alternate days depending on the level of exudate from the wound.

This procedure was developed by the author and Mr RG Ward, Consultant Vascular Surgeon. Aintree Hospitals Trust, Liverpool.

Excoriation

Honey dispensed from a tube can be applied to red, excoriated skin to reduce inflammation, and heal any small breaks in tissue. For dry, cracked and painful skin, honey can be mixed with an emollient or a commercially produced honey with moisturising cream applied to the affected area.

Application of honey

Research shows that the amount of honey required to have a positive effect on the wound is generally felt to be 30–35 mls on a 10 cm x 10 cm dressing (Dunford, 2000; Molan and Betts, 2000; Molan and Betts, 2004; Molan, 1999). However, there are no hard and fast rules and much is dependent on the amount of exudate produced by the wound. A rule of thumb is to use honey as one would use an amorphous gel. Wound exudate can dilute the antibacterial activity of honey and can lead to it being washed from the wound (Molan and Betts, 2004). Nevertheless, honey with an average level of antibacterial activity can be expected to be effective in preventing bacterial growth even when diluted more than ten-fold by wound exudate (Cooper and Molan, 1999).

The surface area and position of the wound will naturally affect the choice of dressing suitable for the wound. Honey soaked into a calcium alginate dressing is often a practical answer to dressing large areas, or circumferential leg ulceration, simply because of its ease of application. It also prevents the honey leaking into the secondary dressing and prevents exudate washing the honey away from the wound bed by holding the honey in contact with the wound.

'Neat' honey applied directly from a tube is very effective but, on some occasions, once the honey has reached body temperate, it becomes more fluid and can leak around the dressing. A wound gel prepared with wax has a thicker consistency and is less likely to leak. Honey from a tube is also useful for cavities.

The topical use of honey can be considered for any wound healing by secondary intention, or acute wounds where there is tissue loss. In the author's experience, honey does not seem to have a positive effect on wounds completely covered in black eschar. However, other users of honey have reported that in those wounds where eschar is present, if they are scored with a blade to allow the honey to penetrate through this area to the wound bed below, the eschar is debrided from the wound.

Some honey and honey impregnated dressings are now available on the UK Drug Tariff, giving the practitioner the choice of dressing and application best suited to the position and condition of the wound. At a time when resources, both financial and human, are at a premium, it would seem inappropriate to suggest frequent dressing changes. However, if consideration is given to the amount of resources that have been spent on a wound that may have failed to heal for months or even years, increasing the frequency of dressing changes to kick start wound healing must be viewed as a positive effect. Once wound healing has been established, frequency of dressing changes can be reviewed.

Allergy to honey is rare (Wood *et al*, 1997). Patients should be routinely asked if they have an allergy to bee stings or bee products. It is prudent to withhold the application of honey should the patient be known to have a positive reaction.

In the author's experience, patients are eager to consent to the use of honey on their wound. There are no reported adverse effects to the application of honey to wounds. There have been reports of patients experiencing pain (Dunford and Hanano, 2004; Wood *et al*, 1997): some transient, and some necessitating the cessation of treatment.

For patients burdened with a chronic wound for weeks, months or years, whose lives and those of their families are frequently disrupted, honey may be considered as a first line management to a problem wound.

The reader should be aware that the only honey recommended for wound management is that which is specially prepared for this use, and is gamma irradiated to render it sterile. Processed honey prepared for consumption is not sterile and may contain botulism spores.

As with any wound care product, honey presented in tubes or dressings should be kept for single patient use only to avoid cross-infection.

Public involvement in health care is correctly increasing, and is often focused on 'natural' and complementary therapies. The practitioner should be mindful of what is available both in these fields and the more traditional or conventional treatments. However, with the long history honey has enjoyed, the question must be posed as to where it sits in this spectrum.

As honey continues to enjoy a revival and the evidence for its use in wound care continues to expand, it is rightfully taking its place alongside its counterparts in modern wound management.

References

Alcaraz A, Kelly J (2002) Treatment of an infected venous leg ulcer with honey dressings. *Br J Nurs* **11**(13): 859–60, 862, 864–6

Bowler PG, Davies BJ, Jones SA (1999) Microbial involvement in chronic wound malodour. *J Wound Care* **8**(5): 216–859–66

Cooper R, Molan PC (1999) The use of honey as an antiseptic in managing *Pseudomonas* infection. *J Wound Care* **8**(4): 161–3

Cooper RA, Molan PC, Harding KG (1999) Antibacterial activity of honey against strains of *Staphylococcus aureus* from infected wounds. *J R Soc Med* **92**: 283–5

Cooper R (2001) How does honey heal wounds? In: Munn P, Jones R, eds. *Honey and Healing*. International Bee Research Association: 26–34

Dunford C (2000) Using honey as a dressing for infected skin lesions. *Nurs Times Plus* **96**(14): 7–9

Dunford C, Cooper RA, Molan PC (2000) The use of honey in wound management. *Nurs Standard* **15**(11): 63–8

Dunford C, Hanano R (2004) Acceptability to patients of a honey dressing for non-healing venous leg ulcers. *J Wound Care* **13**(5): 193–7

Efem SE (1988) Clinical observations on the wound healing properties of honey. *Br J Surg* **75**: 679–81

Kingsley A (2001) The use of honey in the treatment of infected wounds: case studies. *Br J Nurs* (supplement) **10**(22): s13–s20

Molan PC (1999) The role of honey in the management of wounds. *J Wound Care* **8**(8): 415–8

Molan PC, Allen KL (1996) The effect of gamma-irradiation on the antibacterial activity of honey. *J Pharm Pharmacol* **48**: 1206–09

Molan PC, Betts J (2000) Using honey dressings: the practical considerations. *Nurs Times* **96**(49): 36–7

Molan PC, Betts JA (2004) Clinical usage of honey as a wound dressing: an update. *J Wound Care* **13**(9): 353–7

Natarajan S, Williamson D, Grey J, Harding KG, Cooper RA (2001) Healing of an MRSA-colonized, hydroxyurea-induced leg ulcer with honey. *J Dermatol Treatment* **12**: 33–6

Phuapradit W, Saropala N (1992) Topical application of honey in treatment of abdominal wound disruption. *Aust N Z J Obstet Gynaecol* **32**: 381–4

Robson V (2003) Leptospermum honey used as a debriding agent. *Nurse* **2**(11): 66–8

Robson V (2004) Use of Leptospermum honey in chronic wound management. *J Community Nurs* **18**(9): 24–8

Subrahmanyam M (1994) Honey-impregnated gauze versus amniotic membrane in the treatment of burns. *Burns* **4**: 331–3

Willix DJ, Molan PC, Harfoot CG (1992) A comparison of wound-infecting species of bacteria to the antibacterial activity of manuka honey and other honey. *J Appl Bacteriol* **73**: 388–94

Winter GD (1962) Formation of the scab and the rate of epithelialization of superficial wounds in the skin of the young domestic pig. *Nature* **193**: 293–4

Wood B, Rademaker M, Molan PC (1997) Manuka Honey, a low cost leg ulcer dressing. *N Z Med J* **110**: 107

INDEX